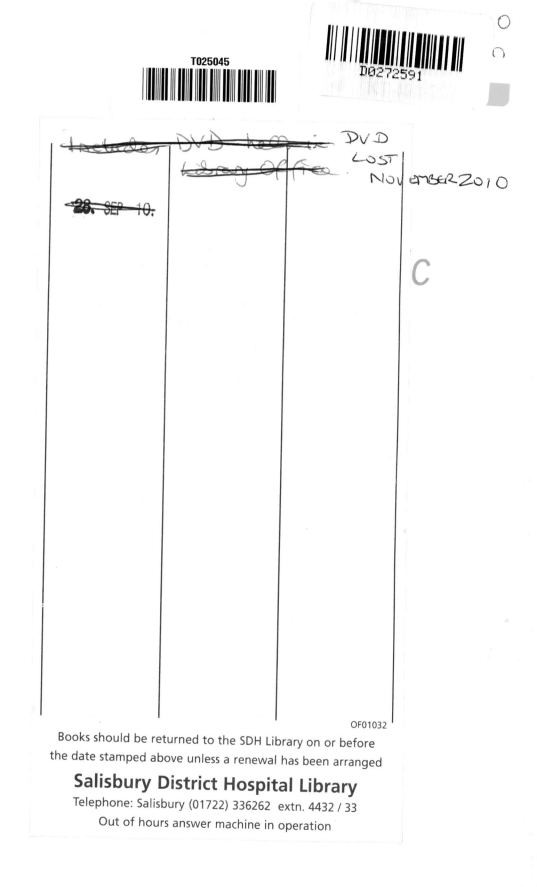

Books should be returned to the SDH Library on or before
the date stamped above unless a renewal has been arranged

Salisbury District Hospital Library

Telephone: Salisbury (01722) 336262 extn. 4432 / 33
Out of hours answer machine in operation

HANDBOOK

Practical Paediatric
Procedures

Edited by
- Ruth Nia Henderson
- Sanjiv Nichani
- Mike Silverman

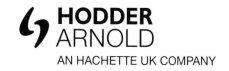
HODDER
ARNOLD
AN HACHETTE UK COMPANY

First published in Great Britain in 2009 by
Hodder Arnold, an imprint of Hodder Education,
an Hachette UK Company, 338 Euston Road, London NW1 3BH

http://www.hodderarnold.com

Hachette UK's policy is to use papers that are natural, renewable and recyclable products and made from wood grown in sustainable forests. The logging and manufacturing processes are expected to conform to the environmental regulations of the country of origin.

Whilst the advice and information in this book are believed to be true and accurate at the date of going to press, neither the author[s] nor the publisher can accept any legal responsibility or liability for any errors or omissions that may be made. In particular, (but without limiting the generality of the preceding disclaimer) every effort has been made to check drug dosages; however it is still possible that errors have been missed. Furthermore, dosage schedules are constantly being revised and new side-effects recognized. For these reasons the reader is strongly urged to consult the drug companies' printed instructions before administering any of the drugs recommended in this book.

British Library Cataloguing in Publication Data
A catalogue record for this book is available from the British Library

Library of Congress Cataloging-in-Publication Data
A catalog record for this book is available from the Library of Congress

ISBN   978-0-340-938799

1 2 3 4 5 6 7 8 9 10

Commissioning Editor:	Gavin Jamison
Project Editor:	Francesca Naish
Production Controller:	Joanna Walker
Cover Design:	Helen Townson
Indexer:	Laurence Errington

Typeset in 10/12pt Goudy by Phoenix Photosetting, Chatham, Kent
Printed and bound in the UK by MPG Books, Bodmin, Cornwall
Text printed on FSC accredited material.

What do you think about this book? Or any other Hodder Arnold title?
Please visit our website: www.hodderarnold.com

CONTENTS

All procedures with ⊙ also appear on the DVD. Please note that some procedures on the DVD have slightly different titles to the corresponding procedures in the book in order to reflect what is being demonstrated in each clip.

Lead authors

Ruth Nia Henderson BMedSci BMBS
DCH nMRCGP
Paediatric Senior House Officer,
Leicester Royal Infirmary, UK

Sanjiv Nichani
Lead Consultant, Paediatric Intensive
Care and High Dependency Care,
University Hospitals of Leicester, UK

Mike Silverman MD FRCPCH
Emeritus Professor of Child Health,
University of Leicester, UK

Contributing authors

Bronchoscopy, Sweat test
Mark Chilvers MB ChB MD MRCP
MRCPCH
Clinical Associate Professor and
Director, Cystic Fibrosis Clinic,
Division of Respiratory Medicine,
Department of Paediatrics
British Columbia Children's Hospital,
Vancouver, Canada

Sleep study (polysomnography)
Priti Kenia MBBS MD MRCPCH
Specialist Registrar in Paediatric
Respiratory
University Hospitals of Leicester
NHS Trust,
Leicester Royal Infirmary, UK

Tuberculin testing
Wren Hoskins FRCP, FRCPCH
Consultant Paediatrician
University Hospitals of Leicester, UK

*Chest drains: insertion and management,
Acute renal failure (haemodialysis/filtration
and peritoneal dialysis)*
James Whitelaw
Consultant Paediatric Intensivist
University Hospitals of Leicester, UK

Resuscitation and defibrillation
Kim Hammond RSCN RGN
Senior Clinical Skills Facilitator and
National Course Co-ordinator
Leicester Royal Infirmary, UK

Mark Fores RGN RSCN MEd
Education and Practice Development
Charge Nurse
Children's Intensive Care Unit
University Hospitals of Leicester
NHS Trust, UK

*Measuring blood pressure,
Echocardiography, Electrocardiography*
Suhair O Shebani MBBCH DCH
MRCPCH Msc Paeds CCST
(paediatric cardiology)
Consultant Paediatric Cardiologist
Royal Manchester Children's Hospital,
Pendlebury, UK

Colonoscopy
Anne Willmott MBChB MRCP(Paed)
MRCPCH
Consultant Paediatrician
Leicester Royal Infirmary, UK

*Blood glucose monitoring, Administration of
insulin*
James Greening MBBS MRCPCH
Paediatric diabetologist
University Hospitals of Leicester
NHS Trust,
Leicester Royal Infirmary, UK

Bone marrow aspiration biopsy
Johannes Visser MBChB MMed
FCPaed(SA) FRCPCH
Consultant Paediatric Oncologist
Children's Hospital, Leicester Royal
Infirmary, UK

Elene Psiachou-Leonard MD FGPA
MRCP(Paed) MRCPCH FGHA
Consultant Paediatric Haematlogist
Children's Hospital, Leicester Royal
Infirmary, UK

Administering medication
James Ian McLean RGN RN Child Dip
HE Dip Intensive Care Nursing of the
Child BA (Nursing)
Matron for Leicester PICU Services
Children's Hospital, Leicester Royal
Infirmary, UK

Testing visual acuity
Lara Abulhoul
Consultant Paediatrician in Metabolic
Medicine
Great Ormond Street Hospital, London,
UK

Hearing testing
Sarah Cheney MBChB MRCPCH
Specialist Registrar in Paediatrics
University Hospitals of Leicester NHS
Trust,
Leicester Royal Infirmary, UK

Julian Anthony Gaskin MBChB
MRCSEd DOHNS
Specialist Registrar in
Otorhinolaryngology
University Hospitals of Leicester NHS
Trust,
Leicester Royal Infirmary, UK

DVD reviewer

Michael Griksaitis DipMedSci
MBBS(Hons)
Specialist trainee in Paediatrics
Northern Deanery, UK

Problem solving is at the heart of clinical management. This has been acknowledged by clinical teachers worldwide. Over recent years, textbooks have moved from a mainly disease-orientated approach, to a more problem-based method of transferring medical knowledge. Of course, as well as clinical skills and medical knowledge, clinical investigation is one of the keys to problem solving and clinical management. Textbooks have not kept pace with the need for learners to understand investigation techniques in detail, in order to become effective practitioners.

Clinical management requires a thorough understanding of a range of therapeutic procedures. Even if individual procedures are beyond the confidence of particular practitioners, it is important for them to have a full understanding of therapeutic procedures, in order to develop management plans and in particular to be able to provide reliable explanations to children and their parents. Of course no textbook can provide adequate training in practical procedures. But a gradual erosion in the duration of training programmes for paediatricians has meant that many procedures with which trainees would have become competent in the past, are now only experienced in theory.

This multimedia text has been designed to address the needs of health professional trainees in paediatrics and child health. The information provided is appropriate for medical and nursing trainees as well as allied health professional students and practitioners. The information provided is relevant to those working in secondary care as well as in primary care and public health.

All practitioners will require competence in some of these procedures, but no health professional will need to be competent in all. When competence is necessary, this text will provide a valuable introduction. Readers will be able to perform essential (core) tasks better after viewing the video and the accompanying script. Many of the procedures will be approached on a need-to-know basis by readers who wish to become familiar with techniques in order to enhance their clinical practice.

We recommend that you dip into the text, rather than trying to approach it from end-to-end. Please watch the video and read the text associated with it two or three times to pick up all the subtle details.

We are grateful to the children and their parents, who agreed to allow us to record the procedures illustrated here. As well as many who contributed to the text, and who are acknowledged in the contents section, large numbers of colleagues helped to facilitate this new venture. It relied heavily on the skills of the hardworking team at OCB, whose technical expertise has enabled us to present the video clips in their current format. Finally, a number of very patient medical publishers at Hodder helped us to complete the complex task.

Dr Ruth Nia Henderson
Dr Sanjiv Nichani
Professor Mike Silverman

LIST OF ABBREVIATIONS USED

AHI	apnoea/hypopnoea index
ARF	acute renal failure
BAL	bronchoalveolar lavage
CSF	cerebrospinal fluid
CSII	continuous subcutaneous infusion of insulin
CT	computed tomography
DCCT	Diabetes Control and Complications Trial
DPI	dry powder inhaler
EMG	electromyography
ET	endotracheal
FiO_2	fractional inspired oxygen
GOR	gastro-oesophageal reflux
GORD	gastro-oesophageal reflux disease
HbA1c	glycosylated haemoglobin
MDI	metered dose inhaler
NCS	nerve conduction study
NIV	non-invasive ventilation
OGD	oesophagogastroduodenoscopy
OSAS	obstructive sleep apnoea syndrome
PAP	positive airway pressure
PEG	percutaneous endoscopic gastrostomy
PSG	polysomnography/polysomnogram
SaO_2	oxygen saturation

▶ Background and indications

Although many paediatricians treat patients with well-characterised convulsions without the use of electroencephalography, neurologists recommend that any individual with a suspected or definite seizure disorder, should have an electroencephalogram (EEG). There are several benefits to carrying out the procedure, including the following.

- The recognition of particularly characteristic or diagnostic EEG features, such as the three cycles per second spike and wave characteristic of true petit mal seizures, spikes originating in the Rolandic area in benign Rolandic epilepsy, hypsarrhythmia and other patterns.
- Presence of features suggesting a focal cerebral disorder such as a tumour, which may indicate the need for specialised imaging.
- Recognition of a generalised cerebral disorder (such as encephalitis) as an explanation for seizures or developmental abnormalities.
- Monitoring response to therapy (although this is more usually done based on clinical criteria).
- Confirmation that episodes suspected of being seizure disorder on history taking, are likely to be epileptic in nature (if for instance an epileptic discharge occurs during the recording); the converse is, however, not true: absence of epileptic discharges on electroencephalography does not rule out a seizure disorder.

▷ Equipment and procedure

A calm and relaxing environment is essential. A period of sleep (natural or hypnotic-induced) is sometimes used to enhance EEG abnormalities. Other procedures which can enhance the likelihood of paroxysmal activity include: periods of hyperventilation of 2–3 minutes and periods of photic stimulation, with a flashing light at 1–50 cycles/s. These are both illustrated in the accompanying CD.

Ambulatory monitoring during which a 24-hour recording is made using a portable recorder may show up intermittent abnormalities.

▷ Different age groups

Infants and young children are generally studied during induced or natural sleep. It is sometimes possible to time an EEG recording during a period of natural sleep for a very young child, otherwise a hypnotic agent (such as chloral) is given. It is important to avoid anticonvulsant sedatives such as benzodiazepines for this purpose. Sleep deprivation on the previous night may increase the likelihood of a period of natural sleep during the recording.

Pitfalls

Since the recording period is usually less than 20 minutes, intermittent seizure activity may be missed. Absence of seizure activity does not rule out fits as an explanation for the child's clinical presentation. About 10 per cent of epileptic subjects may have a normal EEG. Conversely, a small proportion of the normal population may manifest seizure-like EEG activity without any history of fits. During sleep, a number of non-seizure-related physiological changes are seen in the EEG including sleep spindles, vertex sharp waves and others, and should be distinguished from seizure activity.

ELECTROENCEPHALOGRAPHY

▷ **Results and interpretation**

The interpretation of the EEG is dependent on both the technical report (the quality of the recording) and the features which were visible on the recording itself. There are no automated diagnostic methods in routine use. The interpretation also depends on the purpose of the recording (see the section 'Background and indications' above). Some examples of characteristic features are:

- Childhood absence epilepsy (petit mal): 3/s spike and wave with normal background.
- Photosensitive epilepsy: normal background with photoconvulsive spike and wave response.
- Benign Rolandic epilepsy: focal spike discharges unilateral to central Rolandic area accentuated by sleep.

Ambulatory monitoring for 24 hours with a portable recorder may help if the routine EEG is negative or inconclusive. A diary of events, abnormal behaviour or overt seizures should be kept in conjunction with the ambulatory recording, to facilitate interpretation.

Other special techniques include video-EEG recording and special electrodes (e.g. sphenoidal electrodes). Neuroimaging is indicated for several groups of children with seizure disorders, including infants (except those with simple febrile fits), children with focal signs and those with partial or atypical fits.

▷ **Further reading**

Tan M, Appleton R, Tedman B. Paediatric EEGs: what NICE didn't say. *Arch Dis Child* 2008;**93**:366–8.

► Background

The electromyography (EMG) procedure consists of two parts: the nerve conduction study (NCS), which evaluates the velocity and amount of electrical activity along a nerve, and the EMG study. Thus the EMG helps to determine if abnormalities exist in the way nerves transmit electrical impulses (neuropathy) or if there are abnormalities in the muscles themselves (myopathy). It determines electrical activity in muscles at rest and when voluntarily moved (if possible) to determine if the pattern of activity is normal.

▷ Procedure

Electrodes are placed on the skin over the nerve to be studied and they act as microphones to pick up electrical signals. An electrical stimulator is then placed on the skin near the electrodes and is used to create an electrical current strong enough to fully stimulate the nerve. A computer is used to record responses as various nerves are tested. This allows the physician to measure and calculate the nerve conduction velocity and measure the size of the impulse.

Muscles are assessed by inserting a pin electrode into the muscle and recording the muscle response both at rest and with movement. The test usually takes 30–60 minutes to perform.

There are several indications for NCS and EMG studies (Box 1).

Box 1 Indications for NCS and EMG

Common symptoms:
- Weakness
- Numbness
- Sensory loss
- Neuropathic pain

Common conditions:
- Myopathies (congenital and acquired)
- Lower motor neurone disorders, e.g. spinal muscular atrophy
- Neuromuscular junction disorders, e.g. congenital and acquired myasthenia gravis, Lambert–Eaton syndrome and infantile botulism
- Nerve terminal disorders
- Peripheral neuropathy: hereditary motor and sensory neuropathy
- Radiculopathies, demyelinating polyradiculoneuritis (Guillain–Barré syndrome)
- Brachial and lumbar plexopathies and compression neuropathies

---

▷ Nerve conduction study

The NCS measures amplitude, configuration, latency and conduction velocities of motor, sensory and mixed nerves. The conduction velocity is dependent on the diameter and degree of myelination. In newborns the velocities are only about one-half the adult level and do not reach adult levels until 4–6 years of age. A stimulating electrode is placed at two defined points along a given nerve pathway a known distance apart. Supramaximal stimulation is used to ensure the fastest fibres are being stimulated. Surface electrodes record the compound muscle action potential (CMAP) over the appropriate muscle group.

- **Demyelination pattern**: there is reduced conduction velocity (because fast conduction depends on myelin). Patchy demyelination causes attenuation of CMAP proximally but stimulation nearer the muscle (distal to site) gives normal results.
- **Axonal neuropathy pattern**: there is reduced amplitude of action potentials with normal maintained conduction velocities.
- **Conduction block**: this is a feature of acute and chronic inflammatory demyelinating polyneuropathies (i.e. Guillain–Barré syndrome, chronic inflammatory demyelinating polyneuropathy).
- **The late responses**: H-reflex and F-wave are used to assess the proximal segments of the motor nerve function and this is useful in radiculopathies, plexopathies, polyneuropathies and proximal mononeuropathies.
- **Repetitive nerve stimulation effects**: CMAPs are recorded following a volley of 6–10 supramaximal stimulations of the nerve. Changes in CMAP amplitude – sequential decrements – may indicate fatigue of neuromuscular transmission (myasthenia) and in some conditions there is a paradoxical increment in CMAP (Lambert–Eaton syndrome, botulism).

▷ Electromyography

Muscle tissue is normally electrically silent at rest. Action potentials appear with voluntary contractions. Each potential is produced by groups of fibres responding to a single motor neurone. As voluntary effort increases, individual action potentials summate and become confluent to form a 'complete interference pattern' and the baseline disappears. Occasional small potentials are seen if the needle is close to a motor end plate. A loudspeaker system is used to allow electrical activity to be heard.

- **Neurogenic change (denervation)**: the interference pattern is reduced so that the EMG baseline becomes visible. Spontaneous fibrillation potential can occur at rest. These are sharp, biphasic, short duration with low amplitude potentials. High amplitude polyphasic fasciculation potentials are notably seen in anterior horn cell disease, i.e. spinal muscular atrophy. Individual motor unit potentials are either normal or high amplitude, long duration and polyphasic (collateral reinnervations).
- **Myopathic changes**: low amplitude EMG with polyphasic short duration potentials. Sound like 'crackles' on a loudspeaker.
- **Myotonia**: spontaneous burst potentials in rapid succession with waxing and gradually waning. The sound is described as resembling a 'dive bomber'. Tapping the muscle adjacent to the needle may produce a burst.
- **Myasthenia**: decay of interference pattern with sustained effort.
- **Specialised EMG**:
  - **Single-fibre EMG (SFEMG)**: in this study, muscle fibre action potential is selectively recorded from a single motor unit (helpful to measure neuromuscular transmission, i.e. myasthenia and fibre density (muscle spatial organisation) which can be increased in neuropathy). Macro-electromyography is modified SFEMG, and recordings are low in myopathy and high in neuropathy.
  - **Exercise testing**: exercise produces characteristic changes in CMAP amplitude in myotonic myopathies and periodic paralysis.

► Background

Endoscopy of the airways is always conducted as part of a set of investigations in a well-organised unit. It can safely provide important information on both the upper and lower airways. In the past, rigid bronchoscopes were commonly used, but they have been almost fully superseded by the flexible bronchoscope. The only role for a rigid bronchoscope is removal of a foreign body in one of the major airways. The rigid bronchoscope can only be used on fully anaesthetised patients, and it does permit artificial ventilation during the procedure.

Upper airway endoscopy can also be carried out using a short rigid device (Hopkins' rod) or by using a fibreoptic laryngoscope. These procedures are almost always conducted by ENT surgeons, whereas lower airway bronchoscopy is generally the province of the paediatric respiratory team.

Prior to the procedure, a detailed clinical assessment is essential and the respiratory status of the child should be optimised. Antibiotics, physiotherapy, corticosteroid therapy and premedication with nebulised salbutamol (to prevent bronchospasm in those with hyperresponsive airways) may be required as appropriate.

▷ Indications and contraindications

There are many indications for bronchoscopy, some of which incorporate bronchoalveolar lavage (BAL) as part of the procedure (Box 1).

Box 1 Indications for bronchoscopy and related procedures (from Moir A, *et al.* (see Further reading))

Upper airway disorders (may be possible to use awake microlaryngoscopy)
Obstruction:
- Nasopharyngeal obstruction
- Stridor (including biphasic stridor)
- Sleep apnoea

Laryngeal disorders:
- Vocal cord dysfunction
- Dysphonia

Lower respiratory disorders
Congenital abnormalities
Persistent lobar disease (segmental collapse or hyperinflation)
Suspected foreign body
Unexplained cough
Infection:
- Unresponsive to antibiotics (BAL)
- Suspected TB (BAL)
- In an immunocompromised child (BAL)
- Repeated infections (e.g. bronchial biopsy to assess ciliary function)
Unexplained haemoptysis
Failure to extubate in NNU or PICU
Difficult asthma or unresponsive airway obstruction
Suspected interstitial disease (consider open lung biopsy and BAL)

Other disorders
Recurrent aspiration of unknown cause
Post-lung transplant assessment

Bronchoscopy is clearly contraindicated unless there is a definite clinical objective. It is contraindicated in the absence of appropriately trained and skilled personnel, and in the absence of a paediatric intensive care unit in case of complications.

▷ Equipment

A range of sizes of bronchoscope are available, to cover all age groups. The thinnest bronchoscopes, which can be used in newborn infants, are less manoeuvrable and have no suction channel, limiting their use to visualising the bronchial tree. The care of bronchoscopes is critical. Sterilisation procedures have to be thorough, particularly if high-risk infections, such as mycobacterial disease, are suspected.

Most operators use lidocaine spray to the cords after the anaesthetic has been administered. During bronchoscopy children should be non-invasively monitored for pulse rate, oxygen saturation and blood pressure. Particular care is needed post-bronchoscopy during the recovery period (see below).

The most important item of equipment is the operator! Almost all paediatric bronchoscopies (apart from those taking place during intensive care, or in older cooperative teenagers) are carried out under general anaesthesia. Four individuals are required to conduct a bronchoscopy: the bronchoscopist, a trained assistant, an anaesthetist and an anaesthetic assistant.

Pitfalls

- The use of muscle relaxants during bronchoscopy significantly alters the physiology of the airways. If dynamic movements of the upper airway (vocal cords in particular) or the lower airway (trachea and large airways) are important to the diagnostic process, no muscle relaxant should be used, and the patient should be allowed to breathe spontaneously. This is therefore important for suspected movement disorders of the vocal cords, and tracheo-bronchomalacia. The presence of a bronchoscope within the airway may itself reduce the likelihood of airway collapse due to bronchomalacia.
- If BAL is performed for microbiological investigations, then preservative-free normal saline must be used for the procedure. A volume of 1 mL/kg (repeated once if necessary) is administered via the suction channel of the wedged bronchoscope and immediately aspirated. Full and timely appropriate laboratory back-up is needed. BAL fluid may also be examined by cytologists to assess inflammatory processes. Post-bronchoscopy pyrexia or even lung infection is more frequent when BAL is carried out in addition to inspection. Bronchial mucosal biopsy carries a small risk of haemorrhage or perforation (air leak).
- Other complications include: upper airway narrowing from oedema often exacerbated by a pre-existing condition, the complications of general anaesthesia, and aspiration, if children are allowed to drink before the effects of lidocaine spray have worn off.
- Postoperative care is vital. Upper airway complications (laryngeal oedema) are potentially serious, needing nebulised corticosteroids and adrenaline and even (occasionally) intubation. Full monitoring (including an apnoea monitor for those under 12 months of age) is mandatory until fully recovered. The pharyngeal effects of lidocaine spray wear off after about 1 hour and the child may then safely drink.

▷ Interpretation

Where bronchoscopy is carried out as an investigation, the results will be reported as follows:

- functional or structural abnormalities observed by the endoscopist
- results of microbiology or cytology

- interpretation of biopsy material (or foreign body)

These data are rarely diagnostic, but need to be integrated with other clinical information.

▷ **Further reading**

Moir A, Kotecha S, Jones G. Airway endoscopy, lung biopsy and bronchoalveolar lavage. In: Silverman M, O'Callaghan C (eds). *Practical Paediatric Respiratory Medicine*. London: Arnold, 2001.

BRONCHOSCOPY

CHEST PHYSIOTHERAPY

▶ Background

As well as traditional postural drainage and percussion, chest physiotherapy now includes a wide variety of active, technology-assisted methods to improve pulmonary function, especially in chronic diseases. Physiotherapists may also have a role in advising on the general management of acute respiratory conditions in non-ventilated young children, for instance with acute bronchiolitis, even where hands-on physiotherapy may actually be contraindicated. Physiotherapists may have a role in lung function and exercise testing, in asthma management and in the evaluation and management of breathlessness (especially hyperventilation and panic attacks).

In North America, respiratory therapists are professionals who deal comprehensively with patients with respiratory disease, in particular those undergoing ventilatory support.

The aims of physiotherapy are:

- reduction in airway obstruction by, for instance, clearing bronchopulmonary secretions and administration of bronchodilators
- reinflation of collapsed or atelectatic lung
- relief of breathlessness and increase in exercise tolerance
- advice on posture and thoracic mobility

▷ Indications and contraindications

Active, hands-on physiotherapy is indicated in the resolving phase of acute lung disease, and in the management of chronic respiratory disease. It is contraindicated in acute lung conditions such as acute bronchiolitis and acute pneumonia, where the situation can actually be exacerbated. The only situation in which acute illness might warrant active physiotherapy, is inhalation of a foreign body, in the very early phase of management.

During the resolution of an acute focal lung problem, active focal and specific physiotherapy may be required. Long-term stable conditions such as cystic fibrosis require a general approach.

Caution is required in dealing with children with other medical conditions such as congenital heart disease or asthma (when prior bronchodilators should be administered). Particular care is required with hands-on physiotherapy in preterm and other newborn infants. Not only can active chest physiotherapy worsen the situation, but there is a risk of rib fractures in the wrong hands.

▷ Equipment and preparation

A variety of devices are called upon to increase respiratory resistive pressure, to create flutter or oscillations in airway pressure (for instance a positive expiratory pressure (PEP) mask) and in the case of children with neuromuscular disease to provide positive pressure inflation (intermittent positive pressure breathing device) in order to improve the efficacy of mucociliary clearance. Nevertheless, most episodes of physiotherapy are carried out without any equipment, simply by postural drainage, percussion drainage, chest shaking or vibrations, or active cycle of breathing techniques (ACBT).

▷ Variation with age and situation

In children who are too young to participate in active breathing techniques, methods that require no cooperation are used. Particular care should be taken with physical forms of therapy in newborn babies, in particular preterm infants. The majority of chest physiotherapy is conducted outside hospitals and health centres by parents or by older children themselves. Thus, one of the main roles of the physiotherapist is to teach parents and children.

▷ Outcome monitoring

The method of monitoring the efficacy of physiotherapy will depend on its indications. For a child with chronic airway obstruction from mucus or poor mucociliary clearance (for instance bronchiectasis, cystic fibrosis, immune deficiency or ciliary dyskinesia) monitoring may be done by assessing general wellbeing (breathlessness), by estimating the quantity and colour of mucus expectorated, and intermittently by monitoring lung function (by spirometry). During acute illness (for instance resolving pneumonia or severe asthma), improvement in pulse oximetry as well as lung function (by spirometry) would be more relevant. Since physiotherapy comprises one component of a set of therapeutic procedures, it is often difficult to identify its specific contribution to wellbeing.

▷ Further reading

Pike S, Phillips G. Physiotherapy. In: Silverman M, O'Callaghan C (eds). *Practical Paediatric Medicine*. London: Arnold, 2001.

CHEST PHYSIOTHERAPY

► Background

Intubation and mechanical ventilation are frequently necessary to treat critically ill infants or children who develop hypoxaemia and respiratory failure.

▷ Indications

- Any child with significant respiratory compromise and increasing oxygen requirements, i.e. FiO_2 greater than 60 per cent, or an increasing carbon dioxide level greater than 8 kPa associated with deterioration in pH.
- Depending on the ability to monitor the patient and available expertise, non-invasive ventilation (NIV) can be done in a high dependency setting or an intensive care setting.
- Most new conventional ventilators can also provide NIV which is being used increasingly commonly. There are in addition more specific portable ventilators such as the NIPPY that only provide NIV.

▷ Contraindication

Pre-existing abdominal distension makes it difficult to use NIV as it is associated with gastric distension which would potentially worsen the pre-existing abdominal distension, further compromising the patient's breathing.

▷ Equipment

A mask is placed over the nasal bridge and the pressure and flow are adjusted to allow adequate chest wall movement. If the patient has stiff lungs in the absence of lower airway obstruction, it is prudent to maintain an end-expiratory pressure of 5–6 cmH$_2$O to prevent collapse of terminal airways and air sacs.

The treating doctor should bear in mind what are normal respiratory parameters for the child's age, i.e. respiratory rate and appropriate inspiratory time, as well as the underlying pathology when setting up the non-invasive ventilator. The two parameters that are set are inspiratory positive pressure and expiratory positive pressure. If the continuous positive airways pressure (CPAP) mode is used then only the expiratory positive pressure mode is set.

Non-invasive ventilation can also be administered via a mask that covers both the nose and the mouth or via a tracheostomy for children who require long-term ventilation, e.g. those requiring home ventilation for neuromuscular disorders.

▷ Principles and modes of non-invasive ventilation

The objective behind NIV is to provide respiratory support to the patient without the use of an invasive endotracheal (ET) tube.

An ET tube predisposes the child to nosocomial infections by virtue of being a foreign body which attracts bacteria, creating a nidus for invasion of the respiratory tract. In addition, there is always the risk of tracheal injury with an ET tube, although, fortunately, the incidence of subglottic stenosis following intubation and mechanical ventilation is not high.

Nowadays NIV usually refers to positive pressure ventilation delivered without an invasive airway by means of a tight-fitting mask attached to the child's face. The mask is in turn connected to a ventilator, which provides ventilation in one of the following modes:

- *Volume ventilation*: In this mode the ventilator delivers a set tidal volume for each breath. However, patient tolerance is often poor. Imagine having a tight-fitting mask on your face with gas blowing hard at you many times a minute, and then think how difficult that would be for a younger child.
- *Pressure control ventilation*: In this mode the ventilator delivers a set pressure for each breath. In these modes, flow will vary according to the patient's demands and because the volume generated depends on the compliance of the lungs, this is not thought to be as uncomfortable for the patient. The inspiratory and expiratory times can also be set in this mode.
- *Bilevel positive airway pressure* (BiPAP): This is being used more often nowadays. It provides a continuous high flow positive airway pressure that varies between a higher positive pressure level and a lower positive pressure level. In other words, when the patient breathes in, the ventilator delivers a breath with higher positive pressure and during expiration a lower baseline pressure is maintained to keep the lungs patent during the phase of expiration. These devices are sensitive and can detect the patient's respiratory effort, even in the presence of a leak around the circuit. Bilevel PAP responds to the patient's own breathing efforts and cycles between the higher and the lower pressures depending on the phase of ventilation making it more patient responsive thereby improving compliance and respiratory mechanics.
- *Pressure support ventilation*: This is a commonly used mode for NIV. The patient takes a breath and extracts gas from the ventilator circuit, which triggers the ventilator to give the patient a breath. When the patient's inspiration is complete, there is a fall in inspiratory flow below a certain threshold and the ventilator cycles to expiration, during which there is a lower baseline positive end-expiratory pressure (PEEP). When the patient takes a breath, the machine delivers flow, and terminates it when the preset pressure is reached or when there is a drop in flow because the patient has stopped breathing in. If there is a leak, this mode is usually inadequate in which case it would be better to use a pressure control mode, which has a fixed inspiratory time and can therefore compensate for the leak by generating greater flow.

▷ Limitations

If the child's respiratory rate is not appropriate for age, then NIV will not work and the child will require full mechanical ventilation.

▷ Indications for early discontinuation of non-invasive ventilation

- Worsening sensorium levels
- Extreme distress and anxiety
- Inability to clear secretions
- Haemodynamic instability
- Worsening oxygenation and inability to maintain saturations
- Inability to tolerate the mask due to discomfort/pain

▷ Monitoring

Monitoring during NIV consists of observing the effect of NIV on the heart rate, respiratory rate, oxygen saturation, oxygen requirement and if possible arterial or capillary blood gases.

NON-INVASIVE VENTILATION

Helpful hints

- Think of NIV as clever ambulatory mechanical ventilation without some of the problems associated with full-blown mechanical ventilation but also without all its potential.
- The various modalities can be used in acute respiratory failure, but they are particularly useful in children with chronic respiratory failure where NIV is delivered via a tracheostomy.
- Sedating these patients – provided you are sure the patient's respiratory rate is appropriate – can help them tolerate the mask better and might help stave off mechanical ventilation.
- NIV machines should be considered early in the management of respiratory failure.

▶ Background

In the past, peak flow measurement was considered important in the diagnosis and management of asthma. However, for diagnostic purposes, it has largely been superseded by spirometry, because peak flow measurement has a number of drawbacks (see below), is very insensitive to changes in airway function, and provides no means of distinguishing between obstructive and restrictive disease, large and small airway obstruction, and upper (or extrathoracic) and lower airway disease.

Peak flow monitoring may still have a role in the management of asthma. Daily or twice daily measurements performed at home can be useful in evaluating the variability of airway obstruction (which can be helpful in the diagnosis of asthma) and in monitoring the response to changes in treatment when changes are made. Peak flow measurement also has a role in the management of brittle or severe asthma. It may also be valuable for subjects whose perception of airway obstruction is poor, helping them to evaluate the severity of their disease, and to commence emergency treatment in a timely way.

There has been much concern about the unreliability of home peak flow monitoring. Manual chart recording is frequently fictional! Downloadable electronic recording devices have replaced traditional peak flow meters and hand-written diaries.

▷ Indications

Peak flow measurement is most useful for monitoring the response to treatment, either during acute episodes in hospital, or at home when changes in therapy have been introduced. One-off measurements in an outpatient or clinic setting are not useful. Spirometry is far more valuable in this situation.

▷ Equipment

Traditional peak flow meters are bulky, and mini-meters are inaccurate. Electronic devices are probably the most reliable, particularly those with an in-built memory device. Peak flow can be satisfactorily measured during spirometry – but adds little to the information gained from a full flow-volume curve.

A nose clip is not needed. Disposable mouthpieces are required. Children with host defence problems (including cystic fibrosis) should be given an individual disposable peak flow meter.

Measurement in different age groups

Peak flow can be measured in children as young as 3 or 4, but not reliably until the age of 6 or 7.

Pitfalls

- Spuriously high values can be produced by coughing or spitting into peak flow meters. Conversely, false low readings occur if the child fails to take a maximum inspiratory breath before the manoeuvre. Other causes for low readings include glottic closure (grunting) and blocking the orifice of the meter with the tongue. Lack of effort and a breath-hold at full inspiration will also reduce the value of peak flow.
- Rarely, in asthmatic children with extreme bronchial hyperresponsiveness a progressive fall in peak flow occurs as repeated measurements induce airway obstruction. A bronchodilator inhaler device should always be available to treat an individual under these circumstances.
- Quality is best judged by repeatability. If the two highest values are within 5 per cent then the measurement is probably reliable. It is usual to record the highest value of three but to stop after eight attempts, even if a consistent high value has not been obtained.

PEAK FLOW MEASUREMENT

▷ Results and interpretation

Reference values are extremely wide, so that it is unhelpful to try to assess mild degrees of airway obstruction by means of peak flow measurement. Similarly, it is not possible to predict a child's optimum value from charts. This is most accurately obtained by recording the highest value after optimising therapy and giving an adequate dose of bronchodilator. This procedure can provide an optimum value from which an individualised self-management plan can be developed, if needed.

The calculation of day-to-day peak flow variability from twice-daily recordings made at home, has been used in the diagnosis of asthma. It is insensitive, and is not used in routine clinical practice.

Measurements made before and after bronchodilator sequentially during acute admissions to hospital, can help to guide therapy and indicate the appropriate time for discharge.

▷ Further reading

Beardsmore C, Silverman M. Measuring lung function. In: Silverman M, O'Callaghan C (eds). *Practical Paediatric Respiratory Medicine*. London: Arnold, 2001.

▶ Background

Spirometers can be used to measure lung function during maximal forced expiration, and less commonly, during inspiration. This provides information about lung capacity (the vital capacity) large and small airway function (from the forced expiratory flow-volume curve, and its components) and, during the inspiratory manoeuvre, the dynamic properties of the upper airway. Although spirometric measurements are rarely diagnostic by themselves, they have wide application in clinical assessment (Box 1).

Children over the age of 6 or 7 years can generally perform spirometry reliably. Below that age the results are increasingly unreliable (see below).

Box 1 Applications of spirometry

Diagnosis
- Single observations are rarely diagnostic, but occasionally confirmatory, or startling (e.g. fixed airway obstruction)
- Sequential measurements may be more useful (e.g. in asthma)
- In conjunction with provocation test (such as an exercise test, or a bronchial challenge test) to measure bronchial responsiveness

Measuring morbidity
- As guide to management (e.g. comparison of objective function with subjective symptoms)
- As baseline for subsequent comparison – disease progression

Assessing response to therapy
- Very short term (e.g. bronchodilator responses) – acute therapy (e.g. inpatient asthma)
- Long term (e.g. monitoring response of cystic fibrosis or asthma to changes in treatment)

Teaching health professionals
Research
- Mechanisms of disease
- Epidemiology
- Therapeutic trials

▷ Indications and contraindications

One-off measurements may be valuable for diagnosis in conjunction with history and physical examination. For instance, if upper airway or tracheal obstruction is suspected, then a full expiratory and inspiratory flow-volume curve should be plotted, looking for dynamic or fixed obstructive features. All children with respiratory symptoms who are old enough to comply should undergo spirometry at their first general paediatric referral and subsequently as needed. Differences between objective values of lung function and the child's clinical condition or symptoms provide important clues to the relationship between the child or family's perception of illness, and objective physiological measures. Subsequent management will depend on the reliability of symptoms as a guide to therapy. The measurement of bronchodilator response (after an adequate dose of bronchodilator rather than 'a couple of puffs') is important in the management of any respiratory illness, not just asthma.

In a children's chest clinic, spirometry should be routine, before assessment by the nurse or doctor. In a specialist centre, spirometry (forced expiratory volume in one second (FEV_1) in particular) is the technique of choice during bronchial challenge testing.

Where upper airway obstruction is suspected, a full inspiratory curve should be recorded in addition to the maximum expiratory manoeuvre.

SPIROMETRY

There are no definite contraindications to spirometry. Very occasionally in an asthmatic child with a high degree of bronchial responsiveness, simple spirometric measurements may provoke acute airway obstruction. Wherever spirometry is measured, a bronchodilator inhaler and spacer should always be available for this eventuality.

▷ Equipment

For paediatric use, a full recording spirometer with immediate print-out of the volume-time and the flow-volume curves should be available. These are essential for quality control in paediatrics. If spirometry is to be attempted in children under the age of 6, then a computerised incentive spirometry system should be installed. A number of these are available which encourage children by means of entertaining computer graphics, to take a maximum inspiration, and then to blow maximally during expiration for as long as possible. They increase the chances of success. Hand-held devices which simply give a read-out of forced vital capacity (FVC), FEV_1 and peak expiratory flow (PEF) may be used for home monitoring by well-practised subjects, but are not appropriate for use in a general outpatient setting. A means of calibrating the machine should be available.

The experience of the operator is as important as the equipment. Measurements should only be made by nursing or technical staff who are experienced in managing children.

It is unnecessary to use a nose clip, unless nasal escape of air is a possibility (where for instance there are palatal problems or facial muscle weakness). Disposable mouthpieces and an in-line disposable bacterial filter should be used to prevent cross-infection.

Different age groups

For children under the age of 6, a computer-based incentive spirometry system is essential. This sort of measurement can only be performed by experts in specialist laboratories. Although electronic spirometers with printing facilities are essential for hospital use, older children may usefully perform home recordings, using a simple electronic spirometer with a downloadable memory. Children with neuromuscular disease may have difficulty maintaining a seal around the mouthpiece. A rigid mouthpiece incorporating a flange helps to maintain a seal around the lips.

Pitfalls

- Up to five practice blows may be required before the definitive measurements are taken. The main quality control criterion is repeatability of the FVC and FEV_1, since it is highly unlikely that any two substandard blows will give values which are very close. Ideally, the two highest values of FVC or FEV_1 in a series of blows should differ by <5 per cent or 200 mL whichever is the greater. Inspection of the flow-volume curve will also be an important part of quality control. Rapid take-off, smooth descent and completeness of expiration are all important features. (See Figure 1).

- The two commonest errors are failure to inspire to total lung capacity before starting to blow, and failure to empty the lungs to residual volume at the end of forced expiration. If either full inspiration or full expiration are curtailed, most of the spirometric values (including FEV_1, vital capacity and the flows at various fractions of vital capacity) will be inaccurate.

- Monitoring spirometry at home using a small memory-based electronic device has the same drawbacks as home monitoring of peak flow: compliance is poor, accuracy may be lost, and the relationship between lung function and symptoms (for instance in many patients with mild-moderate asthma) is often too poor to be a basis for guided self-management.

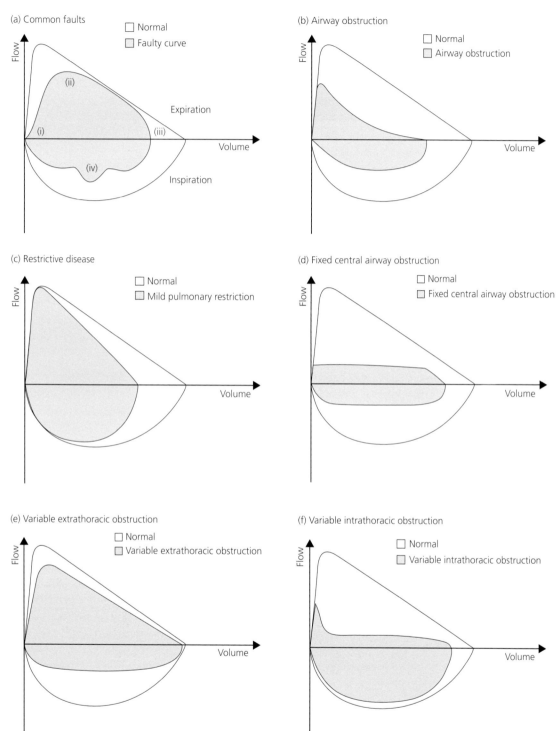

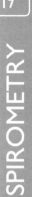

Figure 1 (a–f) Schematic flow–volume curves showing characteristic patterns in some lung disorders. The 'normal' curve (a) shows rapid take-off, a sharp peak flow, a smooth descent to residual volume, and a smooth rounded inspiratory curve. (a)(i) show take-off, (ii) poor effort (blunting of peak flow), (iii) failure to exhale fully before inspiring, (iv) variable inspiratory effort.

SPIROMETRY

▷ Results and interpretation

Remember that there are many causes of a reduced FVC including:

- Obstructive airway diseases which limit the vital capacity by reducing the ability to expire (i.e. 'gas trapping') leading to a raised residual volume.
- Restrictive disorders which limit the ability of the individual to inspire to the normal total lung capacity, such as restrictive lung disease (rare in childhood), weakness of the diaphragm and chest wall and severe chest wall deformity (such as kyphoscoliosis).

The distinction between restrictive and obstructive lung disease is not always straightforward in childhood. Examining the shape of the flow-volume curve can help (see Figure 1), as can the measurement of the bronchodilator response. There are distinctive patterns to the flow-volume curve in the relatively rare conditions of fixed or dynamic upper airway obstruction (such as subglottic stenosis, and weakness or hypotonia, respectively) and fixed large airway obstruction (such as congenital tracheal narrowing). These are illustrated in Figure 1.

Reference ranges for spirometric values have the same drawbacks as reference ranges for height and weight: isolated measurements are often uninformative, given the wide physiological range of normality. Sequential measurements are much more useful, both for diagnosis and management.

▷ Further reading

Beardsmore C, Silverman M. Measuring lung function. In: Silverman M, O'Callaghan C (eds). *Practical Paediatric Respiratory Medicine*. London: Arnold, 2001.

► Background

A polysomnogram (PSG) is a multichannel (poly) recording (gram) during sleep (somno) resulting from a sleep study or polysomnography. Typically a sleep study is done to diagnose or rule out sleep-related breathing disorders, such as obstructive sleep apnoea syndrome (OSAS).

On average children spend half of their life asleep. Respiratory function is more easily compromised during sleep, largely due to loss of pharyngeal muscle tone, especially in active (REM) sleep. Hence respiratory disorders may be exacerbated (e.g. upper airway obstruction) or only become apparent (e.g. apnoea) during sleep. An assessment during wakefulness may mask the severity or miss a sleep-related breathing disorder completely. Such a failure can have an adverse outcome on the child's physical health, behaviour and neurocognitive development.

Obstructive sleep apnoea is common in preschool children with a prevalence in the Western world of 1–2 per cent. A spectrum exists from primary snoring, through upper airway resistance syndrome and obstructive ventilation to classic OSAS. The commonest symptom reported is snoring which may be habitual (i.e. occurring most nights, even without a cold) in up to 10 per cent of young children. A history of snoring accompanied by reports of mouth breathing, restless sleep, abnormal postures, dyspnoea, apnoea and autonomic disturbances such as sweating are important clues to sleep-related breathing disorders. Children with OSAS may be difficult to rouse or be irritable on waking, have morning headaches and loss of appetite. Daytime sleepiness is not as common in children as in adults. However, lack of concentration, learning difficulties and hyperactivity are commonly reported.

Obstructive sleep apnoea is a dynamic process resulting from a combination of structural and neuromotor abnormalities rather than from structural abnormalities alone. Children at increased risk are those with adenotonsillar hypertrophy, craniofacial abnormalities, obesity, chronic respiratory or chest wall disease and neuromuscular problems affecting upper airway and respiratory muscle function. Untreated OSAS can result in growth failure, neurocognitive deficits and behavioural problems. Pulmonary hypertension and cor pulmonale are described in infancy.

Central hypoventilation is rare. It may be primary (congenital central hypoventilation syndrome), or secondary to various causes such as obesity, brainstem lesions, neurological diseases, metabolic conditions and drugs. Other causes of daytime sleepiness such as narcolepsy or circadian rhythm disturbances are not common in children.

Overnight polysomnography is the gold standard investigation for suspected sleep-related breathing disorders in children. Other screening tests such as nocturnal videotaping, pulse oximetry or nap PSGs have limited utility. They indicate OSAS if positive, but have a low negative predictive value.

▷ Indications

There are limited resources for full polysomnography in children in many countries. Thus a detailed clinical history, an Epworth sleepiness score (normal is <10/24) and physical examination are required to make appropriate use of this investigation. The indications include:

● history suggestive of OSA (with a low threshold for polysomnography in children with Down's syndrome and sickle cell disease)

- complex and high-risk groups such as those with craniofacial abnormalities and neuromuscular disorders: when symptomatic or as a screening tool on 6–12 monthly basis
- suspected central hypoventilation syndrome
- investigation of apnoea/bradycardia in children (but not routine investigation of uncomplicated apparent life-threatening events)
- children with bronchopulmonary dysplasia, restrictive lung or chest wall disease and cystic fibrosis who have prolonged or significant recurrent hypoxaemia on oximetry studies

▷ Contraindications

Full polysomnography can be successfully performed at all ages and there are no absolute contraindications. A relative contraindication is a child who does not tolerate the attached wires and cannot be put to sleep without sedation. Sedation and sleep deprivation can both skew the results towards abnormality and should be avoided.

▷ Equipment and materials

Full polysomnography consists of a record of a number of physiological variables measured simultaneously and includes a minimum of 11 channels. More channels can be added depending on the clinical context. Typically the channels record respiratory movements (chest and abdominal wall movements), end-tidal carbon dioxide, heart rate and rhythm, sleep state and muscle activity. Audio-video recording is usually performed as part of the full PSG. Supervision by trained personnel is required and polysomnography should only be performed in specialist centres, in a child-friendly environment.

The setting should accommodate a parent and provide conditions as close to the child's usual sleep habits. Overnight sleep studies should begin at the child's normal bedtime. Ideally 7–8 hours record should be available, but sometimes adequate information may be available in shorter records which include at least one sleep cycle, including a REM (active sleep) period.

- **Sleep variables** collected include total sleep time, sleep efficiency, distribution of the various sleep stages as percentage of the total sleep time (usually REM and non-REM staging is sufficient), sleep latency, number of arousals, body movements, body posture and sleep behaviour (parasomnias).
- **Respiratory variables** collected include the number, type and duration of apnoeas, episodes of partial obstruction measured as hypopnoeas, whether obstructive or central and the frequency and duration of paradoxical inspiratory rib-cage movements with associated desaturation or increased end-tidal carbon dioxide values. Thermistors are commonly used to record airflow but may not reliably record partial airway obstructive events.
- **Non-respiratory variables** recorded include snoring and cardiac rate and rhythm. Videotaping may be useful in interpreting unusual behaviour events and respiratory effort during sleep.

Pitfalls

- **First night effect** is related to unusual surroundings and use of a single night's recording. Usually a single night study is thought to be sufficient to exclude clinically important sleep-disordered breathing problems, but limited data are available on the reproducibility, sensitivity and specificity of a single recording in children.

- Loss of signal during the recording – if technically inadequate, the PSG will need to be done again.
- Size of equipment cannot be adjusted for various ages and may be obtrusive.
- Expensive and time-consuming.

▷ Data interpretation

Computerised data acquisition and scoring are attractive, but of limited use in children due to significant overlap of normal and abnormal respiratory events. The record should be scored by a fully qualified individual who knows the unique characteristics of breathing during sleep in children of various ages. The record is scored in epochs of 30 seconds in children over 6 months.

The specific respiratory events leading to disruption of the normal sleeping pattern are listed below.

- **Obstructive apnoea**: Complete cessation of airflow at the nose or mouth for at least 10 seconds with out-of-phase (paradoxical) movements of the chest (rib-cage) and abdominal wall (Figure 1).
- **Obstructive hypopnoea**: 50 per cent or greater decrease in the airflow at the nose or mouth for at least 10 seconds with out-of-phase (paradoxical) movements of the chest and abdominal wall. OSAS in children may present with frequent or prolonged periods of partial upper airway obstruction (hypopnoeas), rather than episodes of complete obstruction (apnoeas). An apnoea/hypopnoea index (AHI) of >10 suggests severe OSAS.
- **Central apnoea**: Cessation of airflow at the nose or mouth for at least 20 seconds with absence of movements of the chest and abdominal wall (Figure 2).
- **Mixed apnoea**: Combination of central and obstructive events in the same recording.

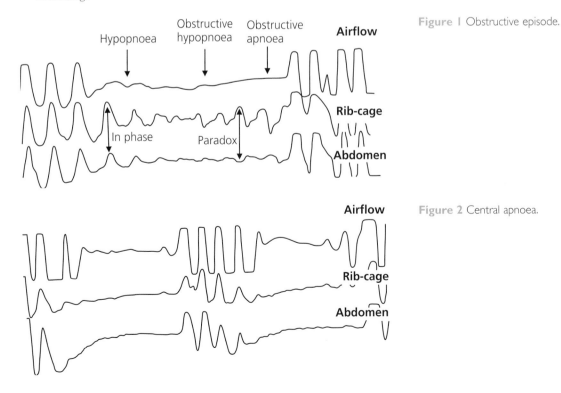

Figure 1 Obstructive episode.

Figure 2 Central apnoea.

SLEEP STUDY (POLYSOMNOGRAPHY)

▷ **Consideration of the different age groups**

- Age-related measurements of respiratory and cardiac rates must be used.
- In infants <6 months, especially neonates, chest/abdomen asynchrony in REM sleep is common, but not normally associated with loss of airflow or changes in gas exchange or cardiac rate. Between 7 months and 3 years the frequency of these paradoxical movements decreases with age. In adolescents, they are not normally seen even during REM sleep.
- Central apnoea without physiological consequences is found in normal children of all ages and is usually <20 seconds, but can also be longer.
- AHI is quoted but not usually used to grade severity as is the case in adults. An AHI >1 is abnormal in children as against >5 in adults.

The recorded data and the clinical details are considered together to provide a report and state whether a sleep-related breathing disorder is present or not.

Box 1 A typical PSG report

A typical report provides:
- Patient's age, sex, height, weight, indication for the study, medical condition and medications used that may affect the study and the Epworth sleepiness score.
- Variables measured, including the quality of sleep-, respiratory- and non-respiratory variables.
- AHI, desaturations, heart rate swings and arousals.
- Possible snoring events.
- Conclusion of whether OSAS or central apnoea is present or not.

Treatment offered to children with sleep-disordered breathing can be monitored by performing repeat polysomnography, if necessary with the patient connected to continuous or bilevel positive airway pressure (CPAP/BiPAP) equipment.

▷ **Further reading**

American Thoracic Society. Standards and indications for cardiopulmonary sleep studies in children. *Am J Respir Crit Care Med* 1996;**153**:866–78.

Marcus CL. Sleep-disordered breathing in children. *Am J Respir Crit Care Med* 2001;**164**:16–30.

▶ Background

Skin prick tests provide a rapid means of identifying IgE-mediated sensitivity, as part of the investigation of a child with suspected allergy. Because allergic sensitisation is common in the population (up to 40 per cent of teenagers and young adults in the UK have a positive response to at least one of the commonly used skin prick test allergens) these tests are of low specificity. Conversely, in many allergic disorders (in particular certain forms of food allergy) skin prick tests may be negative for a number of reasons. Many would say that a careful history, in particular in relation to the identification of ingested allergens, is the most important diagnostic procedure.

The prevalence of atopic (IgE-mediated) sensitisation in children continues to rise in the industrialised world and in urban centres in the developing world. Atopic diseases (asthma, rhinitis and eczema) have also risen in prevalence. A link is probable but not proved.

IgE-dependent mechanisms may be partly responsible for allergy to *Aspergillus fumigatus* as a secondary phenomenon in children with chronic essentially non-atopic airway inflammation such as cystic fibrosis. Conversely, the commonest cause of wheezing in children under the age of 3 years, episodic viral wheeze, is a non-atopic illness within the spectrum of asthma. In a small proportion of children with what appears to be classic asthma, atopic sensitisation cannot be detected. This is similar to the situation in 'intrinsic' adult asthma. IgE-dependent mechanisms could still be operating locally in the airways, although undetectable elsewhere.

Many children with chronic rhinitis fail to respond to any of the normal skin test reagents and may have a non-atopic form of disease.

▷ Indications

The diagnostic process starts with careful history taking. Relating clinical features to allergen exposure is most straightforward when the exposure is intermittent and when symptoms are episodic, causing an acute, easily recognisable response. The diagnosis can then be strengthened using a symptom diary.

The indications for skin prick testing are:

- to confirm that the subject is atopic
- to confirm sensitisation to a specific antigen suggested by the clinical history
- to screen an individual for potential sensitisation to a number of antigens
- to rule out IgE-mediated sensitisation to particular environmental antigens

▷ Contraindications

The only possible contraindication is severe, life-threatening anaphylaxis in response to a known exposure. Otherwise the procedure is entirely safe.

A relative contraindication is the use of oral antihistamines or local corticosteroid creams within the previous few days, both of which can lead to false-negative responses.

▷ Equipment and materials

In the UK, the allergen test solution is chosen as follows:

- *Simply to identify atopy*: house dust mite, cat and mixed grass pollen.
- *For perennial asthma*: add mould mix, dog, eggs, milk, tree mix and cockroach.
- *For seasonal asthma*: spring – trees; summer – flowers and grasses; autumn – moulds.
- *In intractable asthma or cystic fibrosis*: *Aspergillus fumigatus* is included.

- *Anaphylaxis*: nuts, fish, shellfish and other suspect foods (including soya, wheat, egg and milk).
- Other allergens as indicated by *history*.

A negative control (diluent) and positive control (10 per cent histamine solution) are always included, the former to detect a non-specific response to the trauma of skin prick testing and the latter to ensure the potential for the skin to react (and to exclude inadvertent use of antihistamines). Important aeroallergens vary around the world depending on the climate and local flora (Table 1). The potency of allergen extracts varies between sources and manufacturers. Different skin prick test needles produce different sized wheals. It is therefore important to standardise both the source of the extract and the needles for any individual centre.

Table 1 Some important aeroallergens worldwide

Situation	Allergens
Temperate areas	House dust mite (Der p 1)
	Cat (Fed d 1)
	Grass pollen
Urban USA	Cockroach
Desert areas	Alternaria
Scandinavia	Birch pollen
Mediterranean	Olive pollen

The choice of skin prick test lancet is important. A single use, shouldered metal lancet is ideal, applied firmly perpendicular to the skin surface, so that the shoulders meet the skin surface, as shown in the DVD. The principle behind the test is that by breaching the epidermis, through a drop of allergen extract, sufficient allergen molecules enter the dermis to trigger the release of preformed inflammatory agents, including histamine, from specifically IgE-sensitised mast cells.

A wheal (capillary leakage with oedema) and flare (a neural axon reflex causing vasodilatation) results. The mean diameter of the wheal is a measure of the response. The flare is non-specific. Both false-positive and false-negative results may occur (Box 1).

Box 1 Causes of false positive and negative results

False positive
- 'Aggressive' technique
- Sensitised by allergen unrelated to disease
- Dermographism or eczema causes exaggerated response
- Pseudopodia (tend to exaggerate the size of response rather than cause true false-positive result)

False negative
- Child too young
- Antihistamines taken within previous 48 hours
- Delicate technique
- Poor cutaneous expression of lung-selective immune process
- Very high levels of polyclonal IgE (nematode infection)
- Non-IgE-dependent mechanism for allergic disease
- Unreactive site chosen for tests
- Local corticosteroid creams

▷ Response in different age groups

In the population as a whole, the prevalence of atopic sensitisation by skin prick testing increases with age to a maximum in late teenage and early adult life. Very young children often fail to respond or produce very small responses despite sensitisation.

To avoid anxiety in a young child it may be better to perform skin tests on the child's back rather than the volar aspect of the arm.

Pitfalls

Some of the pitfalls are described in Box 1 dealing with false-positive and false-negative results. Remember that non-IgE-mediated allergic responses will not be identified by skin prick testing.

▷ Results and interpretation

The size of the wheal (the average of the maximum diameter and its perpendicular) is a measure of response. A response of 3 mm or more (2 mm in an infant), in the presence of a negative response to the negative control, and a positive response to the (histamine) positive control solution is an indication of sensitisation. This does **not** imply clinical relevance. For perennial aeroallergens, in an asthmatic subject a wheal size of more than 5 mm is likely to be clinically significant. However, because of the high frequency of atopic sensitisation in the population at large, further confirmation may be necessary.

Confirmation may be obtained by more detailed history taking, by a prospective clinical diary, or by excluding the relevant allergen (if possible) and observing the outcome. Although it may be relatively easy to exclude a food allergen, some aeroallergens (house dust mite, cat dander) are virtually impossible to avoid. Negative skin prick test responses in a patient who might otherwise be suspected of an allergic disease (such as a child with severe asthma) raise the possibility of alternative inflammatory mechanisms, or an alternative diagnosis.

Skin prick tests may be backed-up by laboratory measurements of total or specific IgE and where indicated by non-IgE antibody measurements (such as precipitins). Other measurements which may be useful include C1-esterase levels in recurrent angioedema and serum tryptase, which has good diagnostic specificity and sensitivity in acute anaphylaxis. Challenge tests are relatively rarely used and potentially dangerous.

▷ Further reading

Warner JA, Warner JO. Allergy. In: Silverman M (ed.). *Childhood Asthma and Other Wheezing Disorders*, 2nd edn. London: Arnold, 2002.

► ## Background

Despite the advent of genetic testing for cystic fibrosis, the sweat test is still an important diagnostic tool. It should be used to confirm a suspect diagnosis, even if the genotype is known, and to exclude cystic fibrosis where there are suspicious symptoms. Sweat testing should be performed on infants in whom a raised immunoreactive trypsin has been identified on a screening blood sample and confirmed by a repeat test. An experienced operator is required to perform the test to avoid artefacts.

The basis of the test is still pilocarpine iontophoresis. A small electric current facilitates the diffusion of the cholinergic agent pilocarpine to sweat glands via their ducts, in order to induce sweating. Chloride and sodium levels are greater than normal in cystic fibrosis.

Patients with cystic fibrosis have a negative potential difference across respiratory epithelia compared with normal subjects. This is the basis of a further test which can be carried out if the sweat test is repeatedly inconclusive. Nasal potential difference is not universally available and only performed in some centres.

▷ ## Indications

The indications are to confirm or refute the diagnosis of cystic fibrosis. The pulmonary indications include:

- Chronic productive cough or lower respiratory symptoms which are slow to clear following a respiratory tract infection (particularly in infancy)
- 'Difficult' asthma
- Chronic features of malabsorption or failure to thrive
- Neonatal meconium ileus or neonatal hepatitis syndrome
- A sibling with cystic fibrosis

There are no contraindications.

▷ ## Equipment

The traditional method of pilocarpine iontophoresis relies on the collection of sweat on a pre-weighed filter paper placed over the site of iontophoresis with a waterproof seal. When collection is complete, the filter paper is placed in a sealed container and reweighed in order to determine the quantity of sweat collected (>100 mg is the target) before eluting in order to measure the sodium and chloride content. Alternative devices include the macroduct, which collects sweat in a capillary tube and provides an indirect measure of electrolyte level from sweat osmolality.

Different age groups

It is usual to collect sweat from the arm of a toddler or older child. In order to collect sufficient sweat, it may be necessary to collect sweat from the back of an infant. It is usually impossible to obtain adequate quantities of sweat in the first few weeks of life.

Reference values change with age: sweat electrolyte levels increase during childhood so that false-positive values are more likely in older subjects. False-positives are rare in infancy.

Pitfalls

- Inadequate quantities of sweat (<100 mg) lead to inaccuracies in measurement and hence small samples should not be relied on. It may be difficult to obtain sweat in very young infants (a few weeks old) and in children with eczema, or rare forms of anhidrosis. The test should usually be performed on children >6 weeks old (absolute minimum age 2 weeks) and more than 3 kg in weight. There are some rare conditions associated with raised sweat electrolytes, so that caution should be exercised in interpreting results from children with endocrine, renal or nutritional disorders.
- A low yield of sweat can be due to evaporative loss, which will lead to a false-positive rise in sweat electrolytes, and conversely an excessive sweat weight might be due to spillage (for instance of a child's drink) onto the collection site leading to excessive dilution and hence the possibility of a false-negative result.
- Localised burns can occur at the site of iontophoresis, if the pads are inadequately soaked in electrolyte solution, or if the current is increased to the target level too rapidly.

▷ Results and interpretation

If at least 100 mg of sweat has been obtained with due care and attention, then values of sweat chloride of >60 mmol/L or of sweat sodium >70 mmol/L are abnormal (but the latter is less reliable) and are within the range for cystic fibrosis. Borderline sweat chloride of 40–60 mmol/L is suggestive but not diagnostic and requires a repeat test. Sweat sodium should not be interpreted without a chloride result (UK NQAS guideline). Some children with rare genotypes and mild disease may only have mild elevation of sweat electrolytes. There are a number of conditions which cause false negative and positive results (see Beauchamp and Lands (2005) in Further reading below).

Teenagers and adults have a wide normal range. A study demonstrated a statistical increase in sweat chloride for normal children aged 1–12 years, but no increase in children with cystic fibrosis. In normal subjects over 12 years of age there is no age-related change in chloride, while the older cystic fibrosis patients show a fall with age. The magnitude of the changes with age is insufficient to cause any diagnostic confusion if the guidelines are adhered to.

The diagnosis of cystic fibrosis depends on a combination of clinical features (or sibling with confirmed cystic fibrosis) and a positive laboratory test (sweat test, two *CFTR* (cystic fibrosis transmembrane regulator) mutations known to cause cystic fibrosis, or positive nasal potential difference test). If the diagnosis remains equivocal, ancillary investigations may be needed to identify the cystic fibrosis phenotype, searching for pancreatic disease or insufficiency, sino-pulmonary disease and liver or urogenital abnormalities.

▷ Further reading

RCPCH Guideline Appraisal. Multi-Disciplinary Working Group supported by the Cystic Fibrosis Trust. Evidence-based Guidelines for the Performance of the Sweat Test. NQAS, 2003. Available at: www.rcpch.ac.uk/Publications (accessed 3 June 2008).

Beauchamp M, Lands LC. Sweat-testing: a review of current technical requirements. *Pediatr Pulmonol* 2005;**39**:507–11.

► Background

All tuberculin tests consist of an intradermal inoculation of tubercule protein (tuberculin). If the individual has been sensitised to the protein by a previous tuberculosis (TB) infection then a delayed hypersensitivity reaction takes place resulting in local induration a few days later.

The gold standard for this reaction is the Mantoux test, which is the preferred test for individuals who present with symptoms. However, because the technique is difficult and relatively time-consuming, other methods have been developed (e.g. Heaf and Tine tests) which are more suitable for mass screening.

In addition to the tuberculin skin tests there are now blood-based tests to detect immunological memory of TB infection. The basis of these tests is the production of interferon gamma by sensitised T cells when blood is incubated with TB specific protein. Previously sensitised T cells produce interferon gamma, which can then be measured.

It is possible that similar tests will decrease the need for tuberculin testing in the future – at least in the developed world.

▷ Indications

The tuberculin test is used when the clinician wishes to know if the patient has been infected with TB. The usual situations are:

- where the patient has a clinical history suggesting TB
- an unusual clinical presentation where TB needs to be excluded
- where there is a history of contact with infectious TB

The tuberculin test is not affected by TB treatment so if the patient is acutely unwell there is no need to wait for a tuberculin test before starting treatment. This particularly applies to possible TB meningitis or miliary TB.

▷ Contraindications

There are no absolute contraindications to tuberculin testing but the false positives and negatives need to be borne in mind for interpretation. There is the possibility of a very strong response if the patient has erythema nodosum from TB which in itself is evidence of a hypersensitivity reaction.

▷ Equipment and dosing

The volume of intradermal fluid injected is always 0.1 mL. This requires a small volume syringe and a fine needle. Insulin syringes are ideal as there is no need to flush out dead space in the needle.

Doses of tuberculin are confusing. There is an international standard for the strength of tuberculin but in the USA 5 tuberculin units (TU) is the standard inoculation for the Mantoux test. In much of Europe 2 TU is standard and the UK has traditionally used 1 TU or 10 TU (also known as 1 in 10 000 or 1 in 1000, respectively). To make things even more confusing the labelling is usually given per mL, so 10 units per mL is the strength needed for a 1 TU inoculation (as 0.1 mL of fluid is given).

The 10 TU/mL and 100 TU/mL strengths have now been discontinued (as has the 1000 TU/mL used for the Heaf test) so the UK now uses the European standard and the Heaf test is no longer available.

▷ False positives and false negatives

There are a number of causes for false-positive and false-negative results (Table 1).

Table 1 False positive and negative tests for tuberculosis (TB)

False positive	False negative
Successfully treated TB – once the test is positive it decreases only very slowly, if at all, with time	Poor immune response – concurrent infection/live vaccination; overwhelming tuberculosis; immunosuppression (steroids/ cytotoxics; human immunodeficiency virus (HIV); immunodepression; leukaemia, etc.); malnutrition
Booster phenomenon – repeated testing may increase the response	
Previous BCG – unpredictable response	Tuberculin quality – inappropriate storage/dilution/adsorption
Non-tuberculous mycobacteria – cross-reaction with a variety of other organisms	Tuberculin administration – poor technique with s/c or inadequate volume injection
	Reading response – timing/inexperience/bias

▷ Interpretation of results

Reading the Mantoux test is done 48–72 hours after injection and the area should be felt with a finger to measure the diameter of the induration. This is usually measured in two directions perpendicular to each other and the largest value taken. The cut-off value for a positive result is essentially a 'best fit' which separates as far as possible patients with TB infection from those without. This clearly will vary with the population tested. In a clinical situation where the risk is high, 5 mm is usually taken as the lowest amount of induration signifying disease.

The interpretation that causes most difficulty is that following bacille Calmette Guérin (BCG) vaccination. Some guidelines suggest using a larger cut-off (>10 mm or >15 mm) and others suggest making no allowance. The effect of BCG is very variable but it is clear that the response tends to decrease with time after immunisation and is less marked after neonatal vaccination. It will also tend to increase after repeated tuberculin retest (booster effect).

On the other hand, false-negative results can occur if the child is not immunocompetent which may be associated with miliary TB.

In summary, the Mantoux test may be helpful in diagnosis of TB infection but should not override the clinical assessment.

▷ Further reading

Huebner RE, Schein MF, Bass JB. The tuberculin skin test. *Clin Infect Dis* 1993;**17**:968–75.

▶ Background

Transcutaneous oxygen saturation (SaO_2) measurement using pulse oximetry has revolutionised the evaluation and management of acute respiratory disease and long-term monitoring in oxygen-dependent children. Most pulse oximeters work by determining the ratio of red:infrared light detected after transmission through tissues. The ratio is measured many times during each cardiac cycle, and the readings are presented as oxygen saturation. However there are a number of pitfalls and potential artefacts. It is important that these are fully understood, in order not to act on the misleading values (see below).

Values of SaO_2 <92 per cent are rarely seen in healthy children and represent hypoxaemia. Episodic hypoxaemia is defined as a drop in oxygen saturation of 4 per cent or more from a stable baseline value.

▷ Indications

The main indications for oximetry are:

- Evaluation of acute illness in which hypoxaemia may be a feature: this includes acute cardiorespiratory disease, as well as acute neuromuscular disease and depressed conscious level; hypoxaemia may accompany any severe trauma, even if the thorax is apparently unaffected.
- Evaluating the severity of chronic disease: intermittent measurements to determine the impact of chronic disease (for instance cystic fibrosis) and the effect of acute exacerbations.
- Monitoring oxygen therapy: pulse oximetry should be monitored within 30 minutes of starting oxygen therapy, and intermittently thereafter. In children on long-term oxygen therapy (for instance those in chronic respiratory failure) measurements should be made during each stage of the sleep cycle as well as during rest and (for infants) feeding.
- Sleep monitoring: pulse oximetry is an important aspect of sleep monitoring and overnight home pulse oximetry has been used as a screening test for sleep apnoea (see pitfalls below).

▷ Contraindications

Contraindications for oximetry as the sole technique for investigating hypoxaemia are rare but important. In particular, during oxygen therapy, deteriorating respiratory failure (with accompanying hypercapnia and respiratory acidosis) may be masked. An important clue is the progressive need for increasing concentrations of oxygen to maintain a satisfactory SaO_2. One major drawback of oximetry is its inability to detect hyperoxia, with its attendant risks (of retinopathy of prematurity) in preterm infants.

▷ Equipment

Satisfactorily used, standard pulse oximetry devices are accurate to within 2 per cent. Portable battery operated devices are available for ambulatory monitoring. Potential problems with oxygen saturation monitors include:
- Movement artefacts
- Interference by surgical diathermy
- Excessive ambient light
- Malpositioning

- Low pulse pressure
- Use of nail varnish with finger probes
- Excessive venous pulsation

▷ Age considerations

Care should be taken to avoid inadvertent hyperoxia during oxygen therapy in preterm infants.

Pitfalls

There are many pitfalls and artefacts, which should be carefully considered in the interpretation of SaO_2 values obtained by pulse oximetry (Table 1).

Table 1 Pitfalls in pulse oximetry

Potential pitfall	Explanation/implication	Action
False low readings	Movement artefact	Note pulse signal (many machines incorporate warnings)
	Probe position incorrect	Align emitter and sensor; compare pulse signal with trace pulse rate
	Low pulse pressure	Circulatory failure or arterial occlusion lead to artefact
False high reading	Carbon monoxide poisoning	Measure carboxyhaemoglobin and full blood gases
Alarm triggering	Low heart rate or displacement of device	Reassess
Respiratory failure	Hidden hypercarbia	Check arterial blood gas if FiO_2 steadily increasing to maintain SaO_2
Anaemia; circulatory failure	SaO_2 does not inform about adequacy of oxygen delivery	Check full blood gases; check lactate level
Preterm infants	High SaO_2 may hide hyperoxia	Measure transcutaneous or arterial PO_2
Sleep monitoring	Absence of episodic hypoxaemia does not rule out obstructive sleep disruption	Full sleep study may be needed

▷ Interpretation

Clearly the interpretation of SaO_2 differs depending on the presence or absence of concurrent oxygen therapy. Provided the potential for artefacts and misleading results has been considered beyond the neonatal period, pulse oximetry is generally a reliable means of evaluating oxygen saturation.

▷ Further reading

Thomson A. Oxygen therapy. In: Silverman M, O'Callaghan C (eds). *Practical Paediatric Respiratory Medicine*. London: Arnold, 2001.

► Background

Oxygen is a drug that must be administered in appropriate amounts, via a proper delivery system while monitoring the patient and the amount of oxygen being delivered.

The administration of oxygen requires the use of an oxygen delivery system that suits the patient's size and therapeutic needs.

▷ Indications

- Hypoxia
- Any sick child should be given oxygen therapy immediately, while a full evaluation takes place

▷ Oxygen delivery systems

Some of the commonly used devices are discussed below.

Nasal cannula

A nasal cannula consists of two prongs that arise from the oxygen tubing connected to the oxygen supply. The oxygen flows into the nasopharynx which acts as an anatomical reservoir. The fractional concentration of inspired oxygen (FiO_2) varies with the patient's inspiratory flow.

- A maximum flow of up to 2 L/min is used to deliver about 40 per cent oxygen to the patient.
- A flow greater than 2 L/min can cause drying and crusting of the nasal mucosa leading to nasal obstruction and irritation.

Simple oxygen masks

Simple oxygen masks are plastic reservoirs designed to fit over the patient's nose and mouth, secured around the patient's head by means of an elastic strap. Holes on the side of the mask allow for escape of exhaled gases and allow entrainment of room air.

- The FiO_2 varies with the inspiratory flow but rebreathing of carbon dioxide may occur if the oxygen flow is inadequate.
- Up to about 50 per cent oxygen can be delivered via a simple mask.

Partial rebreathing masks

Partial rebreathing masks are similar to simple oxygen masks but contain a reservoir at the base of the mask. The reservoir receives fresh gas plus exhaled gas from the patient's anatomical dead space therefore the combined oxygen concentration of the two permits the use of flows lower than those for other devices, such as non-rebreathing masks, and potentially conserves oxygen use. Up to 60 per cent oxygen can be delivered via a partial rebreathing mask.

- Non-rebreathing masks: are similar to partial rebreathing masks except that they do not permit the mixing of exhaled gases with the fresh oxygen supply.
- A series of one-way valves placed at the reservoir opening and on the side ports ensures a fresh oxygen supply without too much dilution from the entrainment of room air.
- The non-rebreathing mask can deliver up to 90 per cent oxygen.

Oxygen hood/head box oxygen

Oxygen hood/head box oxygen is a very common method of delivering oxygen to neonates and infants. Most hoods/head boxes require a flow of about 6–7 L and up to 80 per cent oxygen can be maintained in a head box. The oxygen concentration will vary depending on the oxygen flow rate, the patient's respiratory needs and the size of the port openings.

When high flows are used a layering effect can occur with the highest oxygen concentrations settling towards the bottom, which is why the analyser to measure FiO_2 should be placed near the face of the baby.

Venturi mask

Venturi mask is a very useful and commonly used method of delivering oxygen. Oxygen flows through a narrow orifice creating a jet effect. As a result of this jet effect, air is entrained through the side port, mixing with oxygen thereby delivering a prescribed, stable concentration of oxygen. This mode is particularly useful when there are no facilities to monitor oxygen concentrations.

Helpful hints

- Use as much oxygen as required but as little as necessary because oxygen is a drug and must be treated as a drug with possible side effects.
- If a child is requiring an increasing or high concentration of oxygen, (greater than 60 per cent) and if there is significant respiratory distress, consideration must be given to mechanical ventilation. Infants and children tire relatively earlier than adults.

OXYGEN THERAPY AND DELIVERY DEVICES

► Background

Delivering drugs directly to the lungs by inhalation has many advantages in the treatment of respiratory disorders. Drugs delivered directly to the airways and lungs have a fast onset of action, reduced systemic effects, and a much lower (and therefore cost-effective) dose. However, because the respiratory tract has a number of features that are designed to prevent particulate matter from entering the lungs, the inhalation route, particularly in uncooperative young children, is often highly inefficient. A number of devices and procedures have been developed in order to 'outwit' the defence mechanisms of the respiratory tract. These include:

- ensuring that the particle size is in the appropriate range for airway and lung deposition (2–10 μm); particles larger than this size tend to be deposited in the upper airway, while smaller particles (1 μm or less) behave like a gas and are exhaled with the expired air
- providing a range of devices which reduce the velocity of the particles at the airway opening to reduce inertial impaction; spacer devices and dry powder inhalers achieve this objective
- encouraging children to inhale slowly from inhalation devices, thereby reducing inertial impaction

The choice of inhalation device depends on a number of factors including the child's age (and ability to cooperate), the situation in which the device is going to be used (for instance home or school), acceptability to the child (of particular importance in adolescence), and cost.

Technical aspects of drug delivery affect the efficacy of treatment, but the clinical effectiveness of inhaled therapy is mainly affected by compliance. Although currently inhaled therapy is almost always used to treat respiratory conditions, the inhaled route may be used to deliver vasoactive drugs, vaccines and other agents. This chapter will deal solely with respiratory inhaled therapy.

▷ Indications and contraindications

Asthma and cystic fibrosis account for almost all of the indications for inhaled therapy in paediatrics, but there are several other uses (see Box 1). Different considerations come into play depending whether therapy is used acutely for severe disease, or as part of a long-term maintenance regimen. For example, in day-to-day use at home a metered dose inhaler (MDI) + spacer + facemask might be appropriate for an infant or toddler, whereas during an acute severe episode of airway obstruction, it may be impossible to administer individual doses effectively, and a nebuliser may be required.

There are no real contraindications to the use of inhaled therapy for treating respiratory disease in children.

▷ Equipment considerations

There are broadly three classes of therapeutic inhalation device:

- MDIs: either manually triggered or breath-activated; with or without a spacer device; with or without an attached facemask
- dry powder inhalers (DPIs)
- nebulisers, either jet or ultrasonic

Box 1 Indications for inhaled therapy in paediatrics

Asthma
- Bronchodilator: β_2-agonists, anticholinergics
- Prophylactic therapy: corticosteroids, cromoglycate
- Emergency treatment of acute asthma

Cystic fibrosis
- Prevention/treatment of infection: inhaled antibiotics
- Reduction of sputum viscosity: DNAse; hypertonic saline
- Secretion hydration: amiloride
- Protease inhibition: α_1-antitrypsin
- Gene therapy: via liposomes or viruses

Immune deficiency
- Prevention of *Pneumocystis carinii* pneumonia: inhaled pentamidine

Dyspnoea
- Inhaled opiates

Immunisation
- Measles vaccination

Treatment of croup
- Nebulised adrenaline
- Reduction of oedema: (epinephrine) nebulised steroids (budesonide)

Inhalational drug delivery on intensive care
- Treatment of bronchiolitis: ribavirin
- Adult respiratory distress syndrome: surfactant
- Pulmonary hypertension: nitroprusside, magnesium sulphate
- Bronchopulmonary dysplasia: corticosteroids

The choice of device is influenced both by patient age (coordination and cooperation), social considerations (particularly where teenagers are concerned), the indications for therapy (maintenance therapy or acute treatment) and comorbidity (such as neuromuscular disease limiting coordination). The range and choice of inhalation device is listed in Table 1.

■ Pressurised metered dose inhalers

Pressurised MDIs release a precise quantity of drug dissolved, or suspended in a propellant, at high velocity and require a high degree of patient coordination. Even when used properly, a high proportion of the dose impacts on the oropharynx and only a small quantity enters the lungs. This maldistribution is accentuated when children inhale rapidly from the device and can be overcome by using a holding chamber (often referred to as a spacer), which both reduces the velocity of the particles and by gravitational sedimentation removes some of the larger particles, allowing the remaining suspended particulate matter to be delivered to the lower respiratory tract. For young children under the age of 2–3, who are unable to inhale from a mouthpiece, a tightly fitting soft facemask can be used. It is important that the facemask makes close contact with the face, so that when the child inhales from the spacer device suspended particles are drawn in, rather than simply fresh air.

Breath-activated MDIs are appropriate for bronchodilator therapy in older children. Although they remove the need for hand–breath coordination, these devices may lead to reflex glottic closure as the cold propellant reaches the pharynx (see Helpful hints below).

Table 1 Overview of inhalation devices

Age (years)	First choice	Second choice	Comments
0–2	MDI + spacer and facemask	Nebuliser	Avoid 'open vent' nebulisers
3–6	MDI + spacer	Nebuliser	Very few children at this age can use DPIs adequately
6–12 (bronchodilators)	MDI + spacer or breath-actuated MDIs or DPI	–	If using DPI or breath-actuated MDI, also prescribe MDI + spacer for acute exacerbations
6–12 (steroids)	MDI + spacer	DPI or breath-actuated MDI	May need to adjust dose if switching between inhalers; advise mouth rinsing or gargling
12+ (bronchodilators)	DPI or breath-actuated MDI	–	
12+ (steroids)	MDI + spacer	DPI or breath-actuated MDI	May need to adjust dose if switching between inhalers; advise mouth rinsing or gargling
Acute asthma (all ages)	MDI + spacer	Nebuliser	Ensure appropriate dosing; nebulise for a set period of time; give written instructions

MDI, metered dose inhaler; DPI, dry powder inhaler.

When MDIs are being used to deliver inhaled corticosteroids, a spacer device should always be used to minimise systemic absorption from the oropharynx or gastrointestinal tract. A spacer device is not essential when emergency β_2-adrenergic bronchodilators are being delivered for emergency use or as rescue therapy. The ease of therapy is more important than any potential risk of systemic effects, since the safety margins are wide for β_2-agonists.

■ Dry powder inhalers
Dry powder inhalers are a cheap and convenient means of administering breath-activated therapies in school-age children. They are not always appropriate for preschool children, since when children blow into the device rather than inhaling, the dry powder may become dampened, aggregated into larger particles, and therefore undeliverable to the lower respiratory tract. In addition, some devices require a minimum inspiratory flow, which may not be achievable by very young children, in order to disperse the particles during inhalation.

■ Nebulisers
These are used much less frequently than formerly, with improvement in MDI and DPI devices. Their main indication is for emergency bronchodilator therapy in asthma, for children who are completely incapable of using an MDI with or without a facemask. Again, unless administered with a closely fitting facemask or mouthpiece, the loss of aerosol may be considerable, with consequent under-dosing. Ultrasonic nebulisers are

INHALED THERAPY

less reliable than jet nebulisers, despite their greater convenience, and should not be used particularly for suspended drugs such as budesonide.

Among jet nebulisers there are a number of technical variations, which increase the efficiency of delivery. These have little bearing in clinical practice since when a nebuliser is being used to deliver bronchodilator, the dose is titrated against clinical outcome rather than a fixed dose being used. This is not the case in cystic fibrosis when an inhaled antibiotic or DNAse is nebulised. An area of active technical development is intelligent dosimetric nebulisers, which generate precise pulses of aerosol.

▷ Variations with age and situation

The choice of device in relation to age is dealt with above. Children should be given some choice of device for use outside the home. It is generally unnecessary to use a spacer device, for instance, to administer rescue bronchodilator therapy to an asthmatic child outside the home. Fairly unobtrusive devices such as breath-activated MDIs or DPIs can be used in this situation.

Helpful hints

- Careful tuition is necessary for every child.
- Parents of young children should be encouraged to make inhalation therapy into a game, or part of a pleasant routine, such as the bedtime story.
- Compliance can be enhanced by giving clear, written instructions to every child and family. Allowing young children to decorate their spacer devices may help. Without expensive recording equipment, it is virtually impossible to ensure compliance outside hospital. Seeking information from children themselves (rather than their parents) appears to be a better way of establishing compliance with therapy, but there are no foolproof, simple clinical methods.
- It is essential for an appropriate health professional (nurse or doctor) to observe every child using each inhalation device that has been prescribed to be sure that the appropriate technique is used.
- It is surprisingly common to see an MDI (even breath-activated devices) misused and one of the commonest clues is the puff of aerosol leaving the device or the mouth after the drug has supposedly been completely inhaled.

▷ Outcome monitoring

Monitoring the process of aerosol delivery (in particular compliance) is difficult. Observation, education and re-education are important. By monitoring the take-up of prescriptions, compliance with regular, prophylactic or maintenance medication can be monitored (although there is no guarantee that the drugs have actually been used). In most acute or chronic clinical situations, the outcome of inhalation therapy is determined by assessing the change in clinical status of the child. Lung function tests (especially spirometric tests) can be used to determine short-term outcomes (for instance, bronchodilator reversibility if any obstruction).

▷ Further reading

Barry P. Administering treatment – inhaled therapy. In: Silverman M, O'Callaghan (eds). *Practical Paediatric Respiratory Medicine*. London: Arnold, 2001.

► Background

Endotracheal intubation is the basic prerequisite to providing invasive ventilation directly to the lungs and defines the beginning of an episode of intensive care or anaesthesia.

▷ Indications

The main indications for endotracheal intubation are:

- Severe upper airway obstruction
- Respiratory failure requiring assisted ventilation
- Cardiopulmonary resuscitation
- Administration of general anaesthesia
- Major organ system failure

▷ Contraindications

There are no contraindications to oral intubation but nasotracheal intubation is contra-indicated in patients with basilar skull fracture, maxillofacial trauma and coagulopathies.

▷ Preparation

Like any important procedure, preparation for the procedure is as important as the skill required to execute the procedure. The following are essential.

Access

It is ideal to have two functioning intravenous lines prior to intubation if possible. However, that does not mean that one should delay intubation in an infant or child who clearly needs to be intubated if a single line is functioning well.

Drugs

Drugs from various categories are required: drugs for analgesia and sedation, such as ketamine or midazolam, drugs that paralyse the child to provide a motionless patient, such as suxamethonium or atracurium, and drugs essential for resuscitating a patient in case of an adverse cardiovascular event. These drugs are known as 'crash' drugs, e.g. adrenaline and atropine.

In addition, sodium bicarbonate is useful in case of a prolonged cardiac arrest, and calcium chloride acts as a cardiac muscle stimulant.

Last but not least, an intravenous port should be identified into which all 'crash drugs' will be administered. For the sake of completeness, have volume expanding fluid such as normal saline or a colloid drawn up in case of a drop in the patient's blood pressure.

Equipment

A Yankauer suction catheter must be used because endotracheal tube suction catheters are too floppy and do not provide adequate suction, particularly if there is thick mucus at the back of the throat. If thick mucus is not cleared properly, the glottic opening cannot be seen and you will not be able to intubate the patient.

Endotracheal tubes that are appropriate for the age and size of the patient as well as one size up and down must also be available.

Laryngoscope blade: two types of laryngoscopy blade are available. The Miller laryngoscope has a straight blade which is able to lift the epiglottis up and open the glottic opening. The Macintosh blade is curved and is used in older children.

A bag and mask, oxygen supply and stylet for the endotracheal tube complete the list of other essential items.

▷ **Procedure**

Head position: In the neonate, the occiput is used as a fulcrum, i.e. the head is extended slightly while in the older child, a pillow between the shoulder blades can be used to facilitate a degree of extension (sniffing position) of the neck. It is worth remembering that excessive flexion or extension will kink the very pliable trachea, and not only obscure the view but will also stop the endotracheal tube passing through the vocal cords.

Turn up the oxygen flow to maximum while preparing to intubate. Once the patient is sedated, bag the child with 100 per cent oxygen for 2–3 minutes to build up an oxygen reservoir in the child's lungs, in case intubation proves difficult, to provide a source of oxygenation to the child until help arrives to intubate the child.

The mouth is opened with the thumb and forefinger of the right hand and the laryngoscope is inserted from the right side of the mouth.

As the blade is inserted, one of the first things that the blade is used for is to push the tongue sideways, out of the way of the back of the throat. This will allow visualisation of the epiglottis and glottic opening.

The choice of blade depends on the age of the child. A straight blade, the Miller blade, is used for neonates and its action is to lift the epiglottis away and open the glottic opening. With the Macintosh blade used in older children the approach is the same, i.e. from the right side of the mouth. Once the tongue is moved out of the way, the blade is inserted in the vallecula, the space just behind the epiglottis. Once the blade is inserted into the vallecula, it is lifted up and away from the operator to open the glottic opening adequately.

If done correctly, the observer will notice the head almost being lifted off the bed – the 'lifting of the head' in this manner must not be done if there is any suspicion of cervical spine injury.

Once the tube is inserted, both axillae should be auscultated for breath sounds. Listening only over the anterior aspect of the chest is inadequate, especially in infants, as sounds are conducted between left and right hemithoraces relatively easily, giving a false impression of appropriate tube position.

Helpful hints

- Once the child is sedated and you are bagging the child, it is worth sucking out the back of the throat before introducing the laryngoscope as it saves time. There is usually a lot of mucus and fluid at the back of the throat which hinders the view.
- If monitoring is available, always use the end-tidal carbon dioxide monitor to confirm placement of the endotracheal tube as perceived 'air entry' can be very misleading, particularly in a neonate, while the tube is actually in the stomach.
- Do not paralyse the patient unless you are sure that you can at least maintain ventilation by bag and mask. This is because if you cannot intubate the patient and are also unable to support the ventilation by bag mask ventilation, the situation may be life-threatening.
- Too much bagging will fill the stomach with air which could inhibit descent of the diaphragms and impede ventilation. This can be dealt with by manually decompressing the stomach or better still inserting a nasogastric tube, thereby decompressing the stomach and allowing the lungs to inflate.
- Atropine use should be tailored to the situation, i.e. if the patient is already tachycardic it should not be used but should be available. On the other hand if the heart rate is relatively low, atropine should be injected to stimulate the sinuatrial node in the hope of reducing any hypoxia-induced bradycardia.

ENDOTRACHEAL INTUBATION

TRACHEOSTOMY TAPE CHANGE

► Background

A tracheostomy tube is held in place by Velcro tape, which prevents movement or dislodgement of the tube.

▷ Indication

Tracheostomy tapes are usually changed daily, or more frequently if soiled or wet.

▷ Equipment

- New tracheostomy tapes
- Scissors
- Saline and gauze to clean the skin
- Lyofoam dressing
- Suction
- Extra tracheostomy tube

▷ Technique

Position the child on their back with the neck extended over a rolled-up towel, to give better access to the area around the tracheostomy tube. One person must hold the tracheostomy tube in place while the other carefully removes the old tapes from both sides of the tube.

The tracheostomy site must now be inspected and cleaned with saline and gauze, and then dried. Attach one end of the new tapes to the tracheostomy tube and pass the rest of the new tape under the child's neck to the other side of the tracheostomy tube. For additional comfort, a Lyofoam dressing (or similar) can be cut to size and placed under the tapes and around the tracheostomy site.

Continue to hold the tube in place and sit the child forward if possible. Ensure correct tension in the new tapes. Two adult-sized fingers should fit comfortably between the tape and the child's neck.

Helpful hints

- It is important that there are two people when the tapes are changed for the safety of the child. One person's responsibility is solely to hold the tracheostomy in place.
- If the new tapes are too tight they will cause discomfort to the child and may cause soreness of the skin. If they are too loose, the tracheostomy tube may dislodge.
- Always have a spare tracheostomy tube at hand.

▶ Background

The orotracheal route is the most commonly used route to intubate infants and children although some paediatric intensive care units routinely use nasal endotracheal (ET) tubes on admission. Some of the reasons for using nasal ET tubes rather than oral ET tubes are:

- Nasal ET tubes may be more secure and suitable for patients who need prolonged periods of ventilation.
- In order to fix an oral ET tube (as shown in the video), the tape usually goes around the lips and the corner of the mouth. That means that potentially, there is a fair amount of movement around the ET tube, which could lead to accidental extubation on the one hand or even the tube tip moving down past the carina into either the right or the left main stem bronchus.
- The mouth is completely free of tubes, allowing the use of a pacifier, which will preserve an infant's sucking action and facilitate sham feeding or even oral feeding in a select few babies.

▷ Contraindications

Nasotracheal intubation is contraindicated in basilar skull fractures, maxillofacial trauma and coagulopathies.

▷ Procedure

The nasal tube is usually 2 cm longer than the oral tube. For nasal intubation, the new ET tube is inserted into one nostril after adequate lubrication with KY Jelly. The ET tube is passed in a backward and downward direction (along the floor of the nose), rather than just backward, which is a common mistake.

Usually if one nostril will not allow passage, the other one will. Force should not be used while inserting the ET tube as this may result in severe bleeding from the turbinates as well as possible trauma to the adenoids.

After the tube is passed through the nostril, the mouth is opened, and with the help of the laryngoscope the tube is visualised in the pharynx. The end of the tube is then grasped with a pair of Magill's forceps, which are angulated in the lower half. The tube is then guided towards and through the vocal cords and then further into the trachea.

▷ Complications

A poorly recognised complication of nasotracheal intubation is chronic sinusitis caused by obstruction of the ostia draining the sinuses. As sinuses are not well developed in infants and younger children this is mainly an issue in older children.

Helpful hints

- Nasotracheal intubation is easy in experienced hands. It should not be attempted unless there is appropriate supervision or if the patient is unstable. In that setting, it might be easier and more sensible to use the more familiar orotracheal route, and thereby safely secure the patient's airway.

CHANGING FROM ORAL TO NASAL ENDOTRACHEAL TUBE

- Often after passing the tube through the vocal cords it is necessary to advance the external and visible part of the ET tube in order to position the tube at the appropriate length. Having the child in the sniffing position provides the best view of the epiglottis and cords.
- Excessive extension or flexion of the neck will kink the trachea and obstruct the passage of the tube into the trachea.

► Background

One of the immediate concerns when managing a sick child is to get some idea of the state of gas exchange and acid–base balance. This can be achieved by using the capillary bed as a surrogate but fairly reliable marker of the carbon dioxide levels and pH of the arterial circulation. Capillary gas measurements are not as reliable a measure of oxygenation, which can easily be determined from oxygen saturation, by means of a pulse oximeter. While interpreting a saturation trace it is important to remember that the patient's heart rate must correlate with the heart rate on the saturation probe otherwise the information could be inaccurate. A free-flowing blood sample can also be used for blood sugar estimation and blood chemistry.

▷ Technique

As you can see in the demonstration (CD Rom), the capillary blood gas is done by squeezing and milking blood out of either the heel or any of the fingers (avoiding the pulp). The big toe is used sometimes.

Studies have suggested that reliability is not affected by peripheral perfusion although conceivably if you had to squeeze hard to get a blood sample you could skew the carbon dioxide results slightly in the upward direction, as a result of venous admixture.

Capillary blood gases are not reliable in the presence of hypotension but in the setting of hypotension, which is a late sign of shock in a child. Under these circumstances, assume the child is very acidotic and give high-flow oxygen and fluid as part of the management.

Helpful hints

- Remember to avoid the finger pulp due to risk of infection.
- In a sedated child the earlobe is a very useful site although it might be frightening to an awake child.
- The earlobe if warmed up will give you what is called an arterialised sample which means that it will provide a good indication of oxygenation as well as oxygen levels and pH.
- Air in the capillary tube will make the results unreliable so the blood should be dripping fairly freely when collected.

VENOUS CANNULATION

► Background

The management of any sick child, requires access to the child's circulation which is achieved by venous cannulation. The normal human has abundant peripheral veins.

▷ Indications

Access to the circulation is required to be able to administer a wide variety of drugs and fluids that are capable of dealing with the various different types of organ dysfunction that infants and children present with.

▷ Sites

The most common sites for cannulation are cephalic, basilic and median cubital veins in the arms as well as the interdigital veins of the hand and scalp veins in the younger child. Barring some notable exceptions, leg veins are less appropriate due to the risk of precipitating phlebitis and greater technical difficulty.

- The cephalic vein in the forearm and upper arm is large, constant and straight and is the most commonly used vein in the arm.
- The cubital fossa is another important site for cannulation and although the vein is usually not seen it is just medial to the pulse of the brachial artery.
- The superficial saphenous vein at the ankle is large, constant and easy to isolate.
- In children less than 1 year, the scalp is a very useful place to insert cannula. This can be facilitated by shaving the child's hair after informing the parents of the need to do this.
- Finally the external jugular vein can provide reliable access and is often forgotten when trying to cannulate a child with difficult intravenous access.

Care must be taken to minimise the risk of local infectious complications which are not uncommon. Therefore insertion of peripheral venous catheters should be preceded by a thorough antiseptic prep followed routinely by placement of a sterile dressing. If peripheral veins are small, visibility can be enhanced by application of warm compresses, using a tourniquet and/or by tapping on the vein before attempting puncture.

▷ Complications

- Haematoma formation
- Phlebitis
- Cellulitis – a peripheral line should not have a dextrose concentration of more than 10 per cent running through it as that can cause phlebitis

Helpful hints

- While inserting a cannula, remember that most veins are not straight and stretching the skin over the vein will stabilise the vein, prevent buckling when the cannula is inserted and thereby increase the success rate.
- After successful cannulation, ensure firm fixation and adequate dressing. Also the limb might need to be splinted in order that the cannula in the vein does not kink every time the child moves.

► Background

Arterial cannulation is done in patients requiring continuous invasive or real-time blood pressure monitoring or frequent determination of arterial blood gases.

▷ Indications

- Children with cardiovascular or respiratory difficulties or both, or failure of a major organ system
- Infants and children undergoing surgery of any of the major organ systems

▷ Contraindications

There are few contraindications, possibly the only one being a child with a gross coagulopathy, in whom it would be better to attempt arterial line insertion under the cover of the appropriate blood product.

▷ Sites of cannulation

Many arteries can be cannulated, although the most commonly used artery is the radial artery. Other common sites include posterior tibial and the dorsalis pedis arteries.

In the setting of neonatal intensive care, the umbilical artery is frequently cannulated whereas in paediatric intensive care the central arteries are often cannulated. These include the femoral artery, axillary artery and, controversially, the brachial artery, even in small children.

The brachial artery is considered to be an end artery, and therefore theoretically there is a risk of ischaemia to the arm/hand if it is cannulated. In practice, however, this happens rarely if at all, and if it has not been possible to cannulate any other artery, the brachial is worth considering as long as the ipsilateral arm/hand is watched closely for signs of discoloration and ischaemia.

▷ Technique

The relevant pulse is palpated and a 24 G (gauge), 22 G or 20 G cannula is inserted at a 30 degree angle at the site of maximal pulsation. The cannula is advanced until blood is obtained and at that point, the cannula is inserted slightly further or 'transfixed'.

The needle is then removed and the cannula is withdrawn very slowly until the point at which the blood seems to gush out. The cannula is held steady in that position and slid into the artery when blood is aspirating freely into the syringe.

Although fairly straightforward, this is a technique that improves with practice. Sometimes during arterial cannulation, it is clear that the cannula is in the artery as blood can be aspirated freely, but the cannula cannot be advanced. In this situation a wire should be passed into the cannula and then the cannula slid into the artery over the wire.

▷ Complications

Distal ischaemia and necrosis can occur as already mentioned, although these events are quite rare. It seems that 'graduates' from neonatal intensive care, particularly ex-prems are more prone to discoloration and ischaemia.

Rarely, arterial lines can get infected, however, it is thought that as blood is flowing freely in the artery under pressure, infection is not as common as in venous lines. Umbilical arterial lines have been incriminated in necrotising enterocolitis although there is no direct proved link.

Helpful hints

- Use a bigger cannula for older children as it increases the chance of successful cannulation and ensures an optimised arterial trace.
- The final arterial trace should be peaked and snappy and if it is not, besides checking the patient's cardiovascular status it is worth checking whether the equipment is working, i.e. the transducer is at the correct level. This is normally the mid-axillary line, which is in line with the right atrium, zeroing the transducer and optimising the trace.

▶ Background

A chest drain is used to evacuate an abnormal accumulation in the pleural space.

▷ Indications

The most common indications for chest drains in paediatrics are:

- Following cardiothoracic surgery
- Pleural effusion or fluid accumulation
- Pneumothorax

Normally there is a negative pressure in the pleura space which helps keep the lungs inflated. Abnormal collections result in the loss of this pressure, leading to a positive pressure on the lung and respiratory embarrassment.

▷ Types of accumulations

Pneumothorax

- Spontaneous:
  - Primary – without underlying lung disease
  - Secondary – with underlying lung disease e.g. asthma or foreign body
- Traumatic open
- Traumatic closed

Effusions

- Empyema – occurs in 30–40% of patients with bacterial pneumonia. *Streptococcus pneumoniae* is the most common causative organisation
- Haemothorax – in Britain most commonly occurs after cardiothoracic surgery
- Chylothorax – most commonly found secondary to operative injury
- Transudative:
  - Results from increased systemic and/or pulmonary capillary hydrostatic pressure
  - Decreased colloid osmotic pressure in the systemic circulation
  - Both of the above
- Exudative:
  - Altered permeability of pleural membranes
  - Increased capillary wall permeability
  - Vascular disruption
- Neoplastic

Tension

Any of the above can cause a tension. As the abnormal accumulation increases in the pleural space the intrapleural pressure rises on the side of 'injury' leading to a shifting of the mediastinum away, obstruction of venous return and respiratory failure. This causes progressive hypoxia, carbon dioxide retention and reduction in cardiac output, eventually leading to cardiovascular collapse.

▷ Insertion of a chest drain

An understanding of the anatomy and surface markings is an important requirement for drain insertion to avoid trauma to the intrathoracic and intra-abdominal organs. In an emergency the second intercostal space in the midclavicular line is used. A more permanent drain is rarely inserted here largely for cosmetic reasons. Drains are normally inserted in the fourth or fifth interspace just anterior to the midaxillary line, which is roughly level with the nipple or the inferior border of the scapula (Figure 1). In non-emergency situations further information can be had from imaging, such as ultrasound and CT scans.

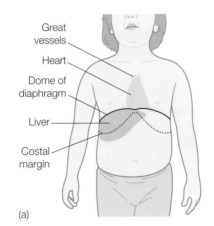

(a)

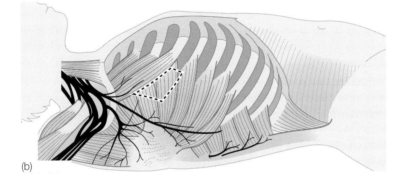

(b)

Figure 1 Surface anatomy demonstrating safe insertion site.

The size of drain is important as a smaller tube is more comfortable with less scarring but is more likely to get blocked, potentially necessitating a second insertion.

▷ Technique

There are currently two common methods used in the UK (Table 1).

Table 1 Comparison of two methods of inserting chest drains

Blunt dissection	Seldinger
Trauma to lung less likely in pneumothorax	Lung may re-expand rapidly onto needle leading to more trauma
Causes more trauma at skin site and more scarring	No large skin cuts
More likely to have a leak around the drain	Better seal around the drain
More uncomfortable to place for the patient	More comfortable to place for the patient

Blunt dissection

Full aseptic technique is used. In the cooperative patient, local anaesthetic is used, but in most children heavy sedation or a general anaesthetic is required as well.

■ Equipment required for insertion
- Sterile gown, gloves and drapes
- Antiseptic skin preparation
- Syringes and needles
- Local anaesthetic
- Scalpel blade
- Sterile gauzes and dressings
- Artery forceps
- Clamp for chest drain
- A suitable size chest drain (8 Fr for a premature neonate to 32 Fr for large adolescent)
- Chest drain bottle and tubing, and sterile water for the underwater seal system
- Sutures (non-absorbable)

■ Method
1. The surface landmarks should be identified and local anaesthetic infiltrated around the site. The best position for insertion is supine or semi-recumbent.
2. The ipsilateral hand should be raised behind the head to optimise exposure of the area.
3. A skin incision is made with the scalpel in the same direction as the intercostal space just above the rib margin. The incision should be large enough to accommodate the drain without tension.
4. A track is now developed through the fat and intercostal muscles to the parietal pleura by blunt dissection, by inserting a pair of curved artery forceps into the wound and spreading them. This may require a few attempts (Figure 2).
5. Before the pleura is breached the drainage tube is kept ready and connected to the underwater seal.
6. The forceps are now taken and held near the tip to prevent their sudden uncontrolled entry deep within the thorax.
7. The pleura is now breached by pushing the forceps over the lower rib using a slight twisting motion and follow the curve of the instrument. A 'pop' is felt as the forceps enter the chest.
8. The forceps are left in place and the grip changed to the handle. The forceps are spread to enlarge the pleurotomy. The forceps are removed and the drain inserted through the track, preferably angled anterior to drain air, and posterior to drain fluid.

Insertion of the drain should not be accomplished with the trocar fully inserted. The easiest method is to partly withdraw the trocar, thus stiffening the drain, but ensuring that the sharp end does not cause trauma to the lung. Importantly in positively ventilated patients the lungs should be deflated prior to instrumentation.[1]

The drain is secured by a non-absorbable suture to form a 'stay' suture. With this technique the same suture that is used to close the skin incision is used to hold the tube. The suture is left long and wrapped around the tube tight and then knotted securely. Alternatively the skin closure suture can be left long and then taped to the tube.

CHEST DRAINS: INSERTION AND MANAGEMENT

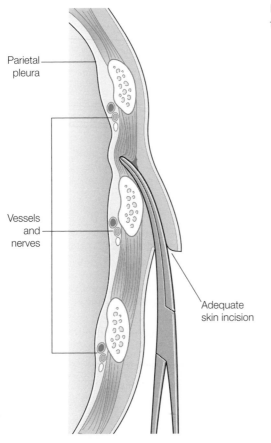

Figure 2 Blunt dissection avoiding the neurovascular bundle.

Parietal pleura

Vessels and nerves

Adequate skin incision

Seldinger technique

■ Method

1. The drain packs come with different contents and thus knowledge of the local product is necessary for preparation.
2. After aseptic preparation, local anaesthetic is infiltrated at the site.
3. The introducer needle is advanced cephalad over the top of the rib at a 60 degree angle.
4. The pleural space is identified by aspiration of air/fluid at which point the needle advance should stop.
5. A guidewire is passed through the needle into the pleural space and the introducer removed.
6. A small nick in the skin around the wire needs to be made and then the dilator advanced over the wire and into the pleural space. It does not need to be advanced to the hilt.
7. The dilator is removed and the chest drain advanced over the guidewire, while always keeping control of the guidewire end.
8. Once a sufficient length of the drain is in, the guidewire can be removed.

▷ Complications

● Infection
  – Pneumonia

- – Empyema
- – Local incision infection
- – Osteomyelitis
- – Necrotising fasciitis
- Bleeding
  - – Local incision haematoma
  - – Intercostal artery or vein laceration
  - – Internal mammary artery laceration (with midclavicular placement)
  - – Pulmonary vein or artery injury
  - – Great vessel injury (rarely)
- Laceration or puncture of nerves or solid organs
  - – Lung, liver, spleen, diaphragm, stomach, colon, intercostal nerves and muscle
- Mechanical problems
  - – Puncture of the lung itself
  - – Chest drain dislodgement from chest wall
  - – Incorrect tube placement
  - – Subcutaneous placement
  - – Intra-abdominal placement
- Air leak
  - – Leaks from tubing or drainage bottles
  - – Last drain port not within the pleural space
  - – Leaks from skin site
- Blocked drainage
  - – Kinked chest drain or drainage tubes
  - – Clots
- Miscellaneous
  - – Persistent pneumothorax
  - – Clotted haemothorax or fibrothorax
  - – Subcutaneous or mediastinal emphysema
- Re-expansion pulmonary oedema
- Re-expansion hypotension
- Recurrence of pneumothorax after chest drain removal

▷ Management of indwelling chest drains

The British Thoracic Society guidelines[2] discourage the clamping of chest drains, which should be limited to changing of the underwater seal and occasionally a trial of clamping to assess an air leak, although there is a risk of tension pneumothorax.

Most patients with a pneumothorax do not need suction, however if the lung does not re-inflate then low pressure suction should be used (2–5 cm H_2O). Suction can be discontinued after full lung expansion has occurred and the bubbling has stopped. The drains can then be removed 24 hours later.

Suction is also used routinely after cardiothoracic surgery to prevent blocking of the drains leading to problems with tension within the pleural cavity.

▷ Chest drain removal

Drains are best removed by two people. One person removes the drain and the other seals the resulting hole. The drain should preferably be removed in full inspiration to prevent air being sucked into the hole. A post-removal chest radiograph should be performed. Small residual air collections will often resolve spontaneously, but the patient must be monitored carefully.

CHEST DRAINS: INSERTION AND MANAGEMENT

▷ References

1. Peek GJ, Firmin RK, Arsiwala S. Chest tube insertion in the ventilated patient. *Injury* 1995;**26**:425–6.
2. Miller AC, Harvey JE. Guidelines for the management of spontaneous pneumothorax. *BMJ* 1993;**307**:114–16.

▷ Further reading

Roberts JR, Hedges RJ (eds). *Tube Thoracotomy*, 4th edn. Philadelphia: Saunders, 2004.

► Background

The intraosseous route is a life-saving resuscitation measure for the short term administration of parenteral fluids. The intraosseous route has a very high success rate and is faster than a venous cutdown and central venous catheterisation routes.

▷ Indications

Intraosseous cannulation is used in infants and children up to 6 years who present with circulatory collapse and/or cardiac arrest when quick access to the circulation is potentially life-saving.

▷ Anatomy and sites of access

Bone is supplied by an artery that then divides into arterioles and capillaries. The capillaries drain into medullary venous sinusoids which then drain into a central venous channel. The needle is inserted into the medulla of the bone which is where the sinusoids are. This technique is mainly used in patients less than 6 years of age. The preferred site is the flat anteromedial surface of the proximal tibia, 1 cm inferior to and 1 cm medial to the tibial tubercle. Other sites that can be used are the midline of the distal femur, 3 cm proximal to the lateral condyle and the distal tibia, just proximal to the medial malleolus.

▷ Method

After antiseptic skin preparation, a standard bone marrow aspiration needle or a specialised intraosseous needle is used (spinal needles are likely to bend during insertion). It is inserted with a rotating or screwing motion. The angle is perpendicular to the bone, directed away from the joint space and the needle is pushed with a screwing motion through the cortex, until a 'give' is felt. Bone marrow fluid should then be aspirated and the needle is connected to intravenous tubing and is flushed with heparinised saline.

Importantly, pressure required to push fluid in should not be any different from that of a patent intravenous line. If it is then the needle is not in the marrow cavity and the fluid will extravasate.

▷ Indications

All fluids and drugs can be given via the intraosseous route. An additional benefit is that the marrow fluid that is aspirated can be sent to the lab to check the acid–base status, electrolytes and the blood count.

Resuscitation drugs such as adrenaline, etc. can also be given through this route.

▷ Contraindications

● A fractured limb
● Any known bony disease such as osteogenesis imperfecta, osteomyelitis or a bone tumour

▷ Complications

● Fracture of the epiphysis
● Osteomyelitis
● Rarely, subcutaneous abscess formation

Extravasation of fluid will occur if the needle is displaced.

INTRAOSSEOUS ACCESS

Helpful hints

- Doing this procedure for the first time can be quite unnerving because of the force one seems to need.
- Hold the needle in the palm of your hand and use a twisting motion to break through the cortex.
- Once in, make sure you secure it very well because mobility of the needle will predispose to extravasation.
- Also use it only for as long as necessary for while it can clearly be a life-saving procedure, it should not be used for the ongoing administration of drugs and fluids because of the associated complications.

► Background

Percutaneously inserted intravenous long lines are widely used in the care of preterm and sick neonates.

▷ Indications

Recommended in preterm or term infants who:

- Have long-term intravenous nutrition needs (necrotising enterocolitis (NEC), major surgical problems, etc.)
- Are likely to reach full enteral feeds slowly
- Have venous access problems

▷ Contraindications

- Skin sepsis at insertion site
- Bacteraemia or septicaemia

Sites

- Large vein in antecubital fossa
- Long saphenous vein
- Posterior tibial vein
- Scalp vein

▷ Procedure

Insertion distance

Measure from insertion site to xiphisternum for leg veins and/or to the sternal notch for arm veins.

Equipment required

On a sterile trolley surface, lay a sterile towel and add:

- Long line set: PermCath 27 G (Vygon)/Epicutaneo-cava Katheter 24 G (Vygon)/ Medex
- 10 mL syringe
- 10 mL normal saline
- Heparinised saline 10 unit/mL
- Needle
- Non-toothed forceps
- Sterile scissors
- Skin prep agent
- Gauze swabs
- Surgical gown
- Sterile gloves
- 2 × sterile drapes
- Steri-Strips
- Clear sterile dressing (e.g. Tegaderm)
- Bandage

■ Procedure

Pain relief/sedation should be considered and used as per unit policy. This will allow relative immobility. If an assistant is required they must wear a gown and sterile gloves.

1. After sterile hand-washing, don gown and gloves.
2. Assemble line (specific for Epicutaneo-cava Katheter): insert reinforced end of line into blue bevel (black marker on reinforcement should be just inside bevel), tighten bevel, flush line with saline, and leave syringe attached to line.
3. Position the infant maximising access, i.e. open the incubator door, slide tray out if necessary and use overhead heater or air curtain.
4. Clean the skin with the appropriate chlorhexidine solution and wait until it dries.
5. Create a sterile field with sterile towels.
6. Apply tourniquet above the site.
7. Position line, syringe and forceps on the sterile field.
8. Insert butterfly needle from the long line set into the selected vein until a good flashback of blood is established.
9. Advance long line into needle with forceps and feed to premeasured distance, releasing tourniquet when catheter is through the needle (the first 5 cm of the line fills the needle).
10. Withdraw the needle gently over the line ensuring the line is stable, by using pressure on the limb above and at the site of insertion. Take care to avoid pulling the line back through the needle since the sharp edge of the needle can cut the line.
11. Detach line at blue connection, remove butterfly needle and reattach connection, ensuring air is not introduced. The black marker that lies over the metal insert must not be visible once connected.
12. Flush the line with heparinised saline. Do not draw back on the line in order to check position. The line will block very easily if the internal wall is coated with blood.
13. Attach the bung and run a slow infusion of normal saline to keep the line patent till the position is confirmed.

For other long lines, the procedure is the same but the line does not need to be assembled, and once inserted, the needle can be peeled apart and removed from insertion site.

14. Secure the line:
    - Clean and dry skin: all blood must be scrupulously removed in order to minimise the risk of infection.
    - Coil long line next to site without kinking and use Steri-Strips to anchor it.
    - Place a postage size piece of gauze under connection to prevent pressure sore and secure everything with Tegaderm.
15. Confirm the position:
    - Confirm the position of the line tip on a plain abdominal or chest X-ray. Intravenous contrast may help in the assessment of the position, and this is routinely used in some units.
    - If the long line is clearly well into the heart or in the liver (particularly if it is curled) and needs to be withdrawn, another radiograph must be taken after manipulation to confirm that it is in an acceptable position.
16. After the acceptable position is achieved, flush with heparinised saline and clamp the line, ready for use.
17. Record in the clinical notes the date, insertion site, length of line inserted and line tip position.

Complications

- Local and systemic infection
- Line blockage and migration
- Rare: cardiac tamponade, pericardial effusion and abdominal perforation

▶ Background

Improved survival of peripheral long lines has been reported for patients requiring multiple or prolonged courses of intravenous (IV) antibiotics, e.g. patients with cystic fibrosis, allowing a more normal and mobile pattern of life.

▷ Indications

Recommended for long-term (greater than 1 week) intravenous antibiotics.

Advantages of long line

- Stays *in situ* for a long length of time
- Avoids frequent intravenous catheter changes
- Can be cared for at home, if medical condition permits
- Reduced chance of irritation and damage to the blood vessels from IV medications
- Reduced risk of infection

▷ Procedure

The procedure is the same as for neonates with few differences. Epicutaneo-cava Katheter is generally used in older children.

1. A good sized vein is identified in the antecubital fossa usually (preferably on the non-dominant limb).
2. Topical anaesthetic (EMLA or Ametop) is used to numb the skin. Nitrous oxide (Entonox) may also be used for analgesia during the procedure.
3. The line is inserted until the 20 cm mark leaving about 5 cm outside for securing to skin.
4. If obstruction is encountered or the line slips out due to the high pressure in the venous system, try: (i) stroking the arm along the line of the vein, (ii) abducting the arm from the shoulder, (iii) flushing while advancing the line. If any sign of swelling or pain occurs then stop.
5. Once the line is inserted to the desired length and is flushing well, obtain X-ray confirmation prior to its use.

▷ After care

- Nurses and parents are instructed to inspect the site every time prior to use and to report if the dressing is loose, wet, bloody or foul smelling.
- Patients and parents are also told to report any pain at the site of insertion or along line.
- Patients are told they can do any activity except rugby, weight lifting, hockey and swimming.
- These lines block very easily and for this reason should always be flushed after use. The flush must be continued until after the line has been clamped off.

▷ Further reading

Beardsall K, White KD, Pinto EM, *et al*. Pericardial effusion and cardiac tamponade as complications of neonatal long lines: are they really a problem? *Arch Dis Child Fetal Neonatal Ed* 2003;**88**:F292.

Reece A, Ubhi T, Craig AR, *et al*. Positioning long lines: contrast versus plain radiography. *Arch Dis Child Fetal Neonatal Ed* 2001;**84**:F129–30.

Millar-Jones L, Goodchild MC. Peripheral long lines in cystic fibrosis. *J Clin Pharm Ther* 1997;**22**:45–6.

▶ Background

Obtaining cerebrospinal fluid (CSF) from the subarachnoid space is the most reliable way to make the diagnosis of bacterial or viral meningitis.

A low index of suspicion is important for children who do not present with the typical clinical features of meningitis, i.e. neck stiffness.

▷ Indications

- Any child suspected of having meningitis.
- A septic neonate or infant and a disorientated older child should be considered for lumbar puncture as disorientation may be caused by meningitis or encephalitis.
- In addition, CSF fluid is important in making the diagnosis of disorders such as Guillain–Barré syndrome, metabolic mitochondropathies and other neurometabolic disorders in which lactate levels are measured.
- A lumbar puncture is also performed for therapeutic purposes, for example intrathecal injections of chemotherapy agents.

▷ Positioning and procedure

The right or left lateral positions may be used with flexion at the neck and hips to widen the space between the tips of the vertebral spines. The lumbar space between L3/4 or L4/5 is usually used.

After cleaning the site with chlorhexidine or povidone iodine, local anaesthetic is infiltrated (particularly in the older child) around the puncture site, and the lumbar puncture needle is inserted.

A 22 gauge needle or larger, depending on the age of the child, or a spinal needle is inserted upwards towards the umbilicus from between the intervertebral space of L3/L4 or L4/L5. The needle passes through skin, subcutaneous tissue and the interspinous ligament after which a 'give' is felt and the needle is in the subarachnoid space. If a spinal needle has been used, the inner needle will need to be removed and CSF will flow. If it does not flow it might mean that the needle is not far enough and will need to be advanced. If blood is obtained, it should be allowed to flow as it usually clears after a while and then the CSF flows. If blood flow persists a different space should be tried.

▷ Contraindications

Lumbar puncture performed on a patient with increased intracranial pressure may result in transtentorial or cerebellar tonsil herniation due to sudden removal of fluid from the spinal canal creating a pressure gradient on the cerebral contents, which can result in herniation.

One should have a very low threshold for performing a computed tomography (CT) scan of the head to try to document the presence or absence of raised intracranial pressure.

It is worth remembering, however, that a normal CT scan does not rule out raised intracranial pressure as changes may evolve over a few hours, but is useful supplementary information when put in a clinical context. Fundal examination is also important but has the pitfall of being very operator dependent, and therefore not terribly reliable.

If the child is very sick, rather than flexing the child into a ball and potentially compromising the airway with the ensuing possibility of hypoxia and clinical deterioration during a lumbar puncture, it is often more prudent to treat the child with broad-spectrum antibiotics and if appropriate antiviral agents, using antibiotics that penetrate the CSF and deferring the lumbar puncture until the child is more stable.

▷ Complications

- Herniation
- Airway compromise
- Infection or haematoma in the subdural or epidural spaces

It is usually a good idea to recommend that the patient lies supine for a while after the lumbar puncture to prevent a low-pressure headache that may be brought on by CSF leak from the space. If this does happen, intravenous fluids to increase production of CSF and analgesia usually help.

Helpful hints

- If whilst performing the lumbar puncture, it is clear that the needle is in the subarachnoid space and there is no flow of CSF, rotating the needle gently without pushing it in any further often facilitates the flow of CSF.
- If you have deferred the lumbar puncture because you think the child is too sick, remember to do it when the child is better because the CSF white cell count may permit a retrospective diagnosis of meningitis to be made. Also remember to do blood polymerase chain reactions, particularly on those children on whom you have deferred the lumbar puncture.

▶ Background

Accessing an arterial line is necessary for arterial blood gas analysis and blood sampling.

▷ Indications

Arterial access allows real-time monitoring of the child's blood pressure and also facilitates blood sampling for arterial blood gases, haematology and biochemistry, and indeed any other serological test that is required. It obviates the need for repeated attempts at venepuncture in order to obtain blood samples from patients.

Frequency of the arterial blood sampling varies with the severity of illness, and the sicker the child, the more frequent is the blood sampling – up to 1–2 hourly.

▷ Technique

Wearing gloves throughout the procedure, first ensure that the three-way tap nearest to the child on the arterial transducing set is turned off to the exit point, thus preventing backflow of blood from the patient. Next, remove the cap from the sampling port of the three-way tap and clean with an alcowipe. Attach a syringe to the port and turn off the tap to the giving set which is connected to the transducer allowing the blood now to flow back from the patient.

Gently withdraw 2–5 mL of blood into the syringe and turn off the tap again to prevent spillage. This helps to remove all of the heparinised flush from the line prior to sampling. Remove this 'waste' syringe and attach a heparinised syringe for blood gas analysis and/or second syringe for blood sampling. Replace 'waste' blood from first syringe if the child is under 10 kg or if the haemodynamic status is unstable, i.e. the child is hypovolaemic.

Ensure no air bubbles are introduced into the arterial line, and thereby into the circulation, by expelling all air from empty syringes prior to use and also by drawing back on the arterial line before returning waste blood.

▷ Considerations

Children over 10 kg: Initial waste blood does not need to be replaced and once accessed, the arterial line must be flushed with heparinised saline in the transducer set using the flushing mechanism.

Children under 10 kg: Initial waste blood should be returned to the patient following sampling of the line. The line should then be flushed manually with 2 mL of saline.

Helpful hints

- Air emboli must be avoided. Ensure all air is expelled from syringes prior to use.
- Arterial lines can occasionally block, dislodge or induce arterial spasm. Carefully observe the arterial cannulation site during sampling and flushing for signs of swelling or blanching. If blanching persists repeatedly the line might have to come out. This is quite common, particularly after neonatal intensive care.
- Make sure the line is flushed well after sampling to avoid blockage by blood clot. That would mean subjecting the child to another procedure to re-site the arterial line.

► Background

Outcome for children who have a cardiorespiratory arrest is poor. The long-term survival rate for a child in asystole without neurological damage is less than 5 per cent. In children in respiratory arrest but in whom the heart is still functioning the long-term survival rate is 50–70 per cent. The best way to prevent disability or death is to recognise potential causes of these events and take preventive action.

It is uncommon for children to experience primary cardiac arrests. It is more common that cardiac arrests are a result of airway or breathing problems caused by injury or illness. Most arrests in children are secondary to hypoxia, caused by some form of respiratory pathology. The early recognition of respiratory distress followed by correct management of airway and breathing problems are vital components of paediatric resuscitation.

Other causes are secondary to circulatory failure often caused by some form of fluid loss; these include diarrhoea and vomiting or trauma causing blood loss.

Faced with a child with a life-threatening condition, a rapid assessment using a structured ABCD (airways, breathing, circulation disability) approach (see below) will help identify problems and alert the responder to get appropriate help. Focus should be on identifying and treating immediate life-threatening problems. Once this initial resuscitation has been undertaken, the cause of collapse should be sought and correct treatment instigated.

▷ Outline of assessment

Airway and breathing

- Effort
  - Respiratory rate
  - Recession
  - Noises, i.e. wheeze, stridor, gurgling, grunting
- Efficacy
  - Chest movement
  - Pulse oximetry
  - Air entry
- Effects
  - Mental status
  - Heart rate
  - Colour

Circulation

  - Heart rate
  - Pulse volume
  - Capillary refill
  - Skin temperature
  - Blood pressure (hypotension is a late sign of deterioration in children)

Disability

  - Conscious level
  - Pupillary signs
  - Posture

RESUSCITATION AND DEFIBRILLATION

The above assessment should take no longer than 60 seconds and once airways, breathing and circulation (ABC) are stable or have been stabilised then management of the underlying condition can continue. Any change in the child's condition should trigger the responder to reassess using the same approach.

▷ Age definitions

For the purpose of resuscitation:

- An infant is a child who appears to be under 1 year of age.
- A child is someone who appears to be between 1 year and puberty.

▷ Equipment and materials

If it is anticipated that a child may require resuscitation then prior preparation for such an emergency can help in the initial management of this event. For example ensuring appropriate personnel are present and relevant equipment (see list below) is available to deal with paediatric emergencies. Each hospital trust will have a list of equipment for resuscitation. It is important you familiarise yourself with the equipment used in your area.

Equipment

- Defibrillator/monitor
- Endotracheal tubes (various sizes)
- Intravenous cannula (various sizes)
- Resuscitation drugs (e.g. adrenaline, buffers, fluids)
- Laryngoscope with various-sized blades
- Fluids (e.g. 0.9 per cent normal saline, Gelofusin (gelatin with electrolytes), 10 per cent dextrose)
- Needles (various sizes)
- Oxygen
- Bag valve mask device
- Oral airways (various sizes)
- Intraosseous needles (various sizes)
- Suction equipment
- Nasogastric tubes
- Syringes (various sizes)
- Giving sets
- Broselow tape

▷ Assessment of the child's weight

Most interventions undertaken during paediatric resuscitation attempts are dependent on the child's weight. However, in an emergency situation it may be impractical to weigh the child. The child's weight may be estimated by one of a number of methods. A Broselow tape relates the length of the child to their ideal body weight. The tape is laid next to the child and the estimated weight is read from the specific measurement on the tape. If the child's age is known then an approximation of weight can be determined using the following formula for children between 1 and 10 years:

Weight (kg) = (age in years + 4) × 2

▷ Procedures

In cardiorespiratory arrest the initial management is basic life support followed by advanced life support.

Basic life support

■ A – Airway

- Open and maintain a clear airway

■ B – Breathing

- Provide rescue breathing (ideally by using a bag-valve-mask device with high FiO_2)

■ C – Circulation

- Provide chest compressions to support circulation
- Ensure prompt vascular access
- Place on monitor to evaluate cardiac rhythm

Cardiac rhythms requiring advanced life support

■ Non-shockable rhythms

- Asystole
- Pulseless electrical activity (PEA)

■ Shockable rhythms

- Ventricular fibrillation (VF)
- Pulseless ventricular tachycardia (VT)

If defibrillation is required (VF, pulseless VT) then it should be instituted promptly and safely. Recommended energy requirement is 4 J/kg.

Drugs and fluids used in paediatric resuscitation

■ Adrenaline

In cardiorespiratory arrest, vasoconstriction is the most important pharmacological action of adrenaline as this increases coronary perfusion thus aiding oxygen delivery to the heart during chest compressions. Dose in advanced life support: 0.1 mL/kg of 1:10 000 solution (10 μg/kg) (via intravenous or intraosseous route). Each dose should be followed by a 2–5 mL normal saline flush. Note: the tracheal route is no longer recommended but if used higher doses of up to 100 μg/kg, it may be required.

■ Fluids

- Fluids are administered in resuscitation to restore circulating volume and ensure that vital organs are adequately perfused.
- Fluids (crystalloids or colloids) are generally administered as a 10–20 mL/kg bolus via the intravenous or intraosseous route. The child's ABC status must be reassessed following each intervention. The underlying cause for a child requiring fluid replacement must be found and treated where possible.

Intubation

The most effective way of maintaining the airway, preventing aspiration, gastric inflation and controlling ventilation pressures is via tracheal intubation. It may also be required for increased effort of breathing leading to exhaustion, severe obstruction of the upper airway, tracheal suctioning or if there is a need for mechanical ventilation. However, intubation is not a priority skill for all healthcare professionals. The priority is to ensure adequate oxygenation and this can be effectively maintained with a bag-valve-mask device, until a practitioner with appropriate experience of advanced paediatric airway management arrives.

RESUSCITATION AND DEFIBRILLATION

RESUSCITATION AND DEFIBRILLATION

Tracheal tubes

The use of un-cuffed tubes is preferred by most hospital clinicians for those children less than 8 years due to the cricoid ring being the narrowest part of the airway.

■ Size of tube

Internal diameter in millimetres is the method used to size tracheal tubes.

- Term infants: 3.0–3.5
- Infants less than 1 year: 4.0–4.5
- Children over 1 year: age (years)/4 + 4

Once an internal diameter tube has been chosen then the length of the tube can be estimated to ensure correct placement. This can be done using the following measurements:

- For oral insertion: age (years)/2 + 12
- For nasal insertion: age (years)/2 + 15

Prior to intubation, preoxygenation with 100 per cent oxygen should be performed. Attempts to intubate should be limited to 30 seconds. If this is not achieved, resume bag-valve-mask ventilation and call for someone experienced in paediatric intubation.

▷ Further reading

Advanced Paediatric Life Support, The Practical Approach, 4th edn. Oxford: Blackwell Publishing. www.ALSG.org.uk

European Resuscitation Council. *European Paediatric Life Support,* 2nd edn. European Resuscitation Council, 2006. www.resus.org.uk

► **Background**

The journey from the operating theatre to the intensive care unit, once major surgery has been completed, requires extremely careful management and monitoring to ensure that the child does not destabilise in transit.

Care of the neonate or child in transit should be equivalent to that provided in the intensive care unit. The child should be monitored to the same degree as they had been in theatre particularly because lighting can be so variable in lifts and corridors. This consists of clinical observation in addition to the monitoring that was ongoing in theatre.

▷ **Equipment**

- Razor sharp vision
- A keen pair of eyes
- Good observation

Monitoring of saturation and heart rate, invasive blood pressure and, if possible, end tidal carbon dioxide levels is a must in any child who has had major surgery.

Drugs

- Anaesthetic drugs should be available to administer if the child suddenly wakes up and behaves in a dangerous or inappropriate manner.
- Resuscitation or crash drugs as well as a volume expander to administer if there is a deterioration in the patient's clinical condition.

In addition to having the drugs available, an intravenous port should be ready to use to infuse the drugs in case of sudden need.

▷ **The next step**

Once you have successfully moved the patient through a corridor and/or a lift, the next milestone in the intensive care unit is a thorough handover from the anaesthetist and the surgical team.

The anaesthetist will have been providing intensive care for the patient over the previous period and usually have assessed the haemodynamic parameters, filling pressures and acid-base status. The anaesthetic sheet usually provides a wealth of information about the airway and drug and anaesthetic use.

The surgeon's account and diagram of the operation performed is useful to help prepare for potential problems after surgery.

Helpful hint

The child is at their most vulnerable early in the postoperative phase and can be set back considerably if monitoring is incomplete.

TRANSFER OF THE PATIENT FROM SURGERY TO THE ICU

▶ **Background**

Accurate measurement of blood pressure (BP) should be part of the physical examination of children whenever possible and appropriate. This should follow the guidelines and recommendations set out by special task force of the American Heart Association (see Further reading). Because the procedure is uncomfortable, measurement conditions are especially important.

Proper training, positioning of the patient and selection of cuff size are all essential. Other essential conditions include a quiet, relaxed environment and a few minutes of rest prior to measurement.

It is increasingly recognised that clinic measurements correlate poorly with BP measured in other settings. 24-hour ambulatory monitoring gives a better prediction of risk than clinic measurements and avoids 'white-coat' hypertension. There is evidence that failure of the BP to fall during the night may be associated with increased risk of hypertension.

▷ **Indications**

Measurement of BP is part of the routine assessment of all children with actual or suspected systemic (especially renal) or cardiac disease, as well as monitoring in intensive care and acute settings.

▷ **Methods of BP measurement**

Auscultatory method

Over the past 100 years the Korotkoff technique for BP measurement has continued to be used despite its limitations. The brachial artery is occluded by a cuff placed around the upper arm and inflated to above systolic pressure. As the cuff is gradually deflated, pulsatile blood flow is re-established and accompanied by sounds that can be detected by a stethoscope held over the artery just below the cuff. Traditionally the sounds were classified as five phases:

- Phase I: appearance of clear tapping sounds corresponding to the appearance of palpable pulse; this is the systolic pressure
- Phase II: sounds become softer and longer
- Phase III: sounds become crisper and louder
- Phase IV: sounds become muffled and softer
- Phase V: sounds disappear completely; this is the diastolic pressure

Oscillometric technique

This was first demonstrated in 1876. When the oscillations of pressure in a sphygmomanometer cuff are recorded during gradual deflation, the point of maximal oscillation corresponds to the mean intra-arterial pressure. The limitation of this technique is that the systolic and diastolic pressures can only be estimated indirectly according to some empirically derived algorithm. The advantage is that no transducer needs to be placed over the brachial artery. This method has been used successfully in intensive care settings, ambulatory BP monitoring and home monitoring.

Ultrasound technique

In this technique an ultrasound transmitter and receiver are placed over the brachial artery under a sphygmomanometer cuff. As the cuff is inflated the movement of the arterial wall at systolic pressure causes a Doppler phase shift in the reflected ultrasound, and diastolic pressure is recorded as the point at which diminution of arterial motion occurs. Another variation of this method detects the onset of blood flow, which has been found to be of particular value for measuring systolic pressure in infants and children.

▷ Equipment

The ideal cuff should have a bladder length that is 80 per cent and a width that is at least 40 per cent of arm circumference (length–width ratio of 2:1). Individual cuffs should be labelled with the ranges of arm circumferences, to which they can be correctly applied:

- Newborn – premature infants cuff size: 4×8 cm
- Infants cuff size: 6×12 cm
- Older children cuff size: 9×18 cm
- Standard and large adult cuffs
- A thigh cuff for leg blood pressure and for use in children with very large arms should also be available

▷ Important points for clinical blood pressure measurement in children

- The patient should be seated comfortably with the back supported and the upper arm bared without constructive clothing. The legs should not be crossed.
- The arm should be supported at heart level, the cuff bladder should encircle at least 80 per cent of the arm circumference.
- The cuff should be deflated at 2–3 mmHg and first and last audible sounds should be taken as systolic and diastolic pressures.
- A minimum of two readings should be taken at least 1 minute apart and averaged.
- In acute care, oscillometric devices are used which give accurate measurement of mean arterial pressure but are often inaccurate for registering systolic and diastolic pressures.
- Postural changes in blood pressure are believed by some to be useful in the investigation of children subject to fainting. Postural hypotension may be confirmed by the failure of the systolic blood pressure to rise when the subject moves from supine to standing.
- Hypertension should be diagnosed only after consistently high values have been observed on repeated visits, or after 24-hour ambulatory recording. Blood pressure should be measured in all four limbs.

▷ Confirmed reference values (Figure 1 and Table 1)

Table 1 Blood pressure levels (systolic/diastolic (mean)) in mmHg by Dinamap monitor in children up to 5 years

Age	Population mean	90th centile	95th centile
1–3 days	64/41 (50)	75/49 (59)	78/52 (62)
1 month to 2 years	95/58 (72)	106/68 (83)	110/71 (86)
2–5 years	101/57 (74)	112/66 (82)	115/68 (85)

Source: Park and Menard, *Am J Dis Child* 1989;**143**:860–4.
Reference values for older children and young people are given in Figure 1.

Practical Paediatric Procedures

MEASURING BLOOD PRESSURE

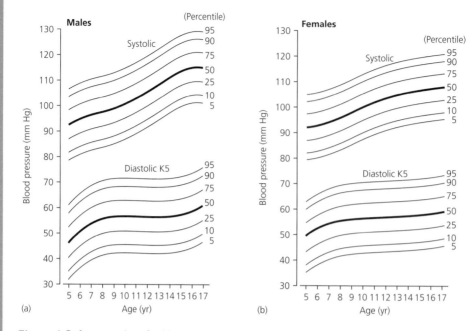

Figure 1 Reference values for blood pressure in children and young people. Redrawn from Park and Menard, *Am J Dis Child* 1989;**143**:860–4.

▷ Further reading

Pickering TG, Hall JE, Appel LJ, *et al.* Recommendations for blood pressure measurement in humans and experimental animals, part 1: blood pressure measurement in humans – a statement for professionals from the Subcommittee of Professional and Public Education of the American Heart Association Council on High Blood Pressure Research. *Hypertension* 2005;**45**:142–61.

Park MK, Menard SM. Normative oscillometric blood pressure values in the first 5 years in an office setting. *Am J Dis Child* 1989;**143**:860–4.

▶ Background

Echocardiography is an indispensable tool in the diagnosis and management of cardiac disease in the fetus, throughout childhood and beyond. It can be used to delineate anatomy (e.g. in suspected congenital heart disease), cardiac function (e.g. in suspected cardiomyopathy) and cardiac involvement in generalised genetic and systemic disorders (such as Duchenne's muscular dystrophy and rheumatic fever, respectively). It is a safe imaging modality with no radiation risk.

Ultrasound waves propagated from the transducers at certain frequencies pass through tissues and are reflected back as acoustic energy (echoes) and transformed to electrical energy by piezo-electric transducers. The signal is then amplified, processed and prepared by the ultrasound machine for visual display.

▷ Equipment

Echocardiography machines have traditionally been cumbersome, although mobile on a trolley. A mobile laptop version is now available, which is easy to use, light weight and small in size so that it can be used in busy intensive care, neonatal units and in outreach clinics. The ultrasound probes are graded in mega Hertz (MHz) – for neonates 10 MHz and 12 MHz probes are used, for infants 7 MHz and in older children and young adults 5 MHz and 3 MHz.

There are several modalities: fetal, transthoracic, transoesophageal, intracardiac, stress echocardiography, contrast echocardiography. In this chapter we will concentrate on the conventional transthoracic modality.

There are several modes: M-mode, two-dimensional (2-D), pulsed Doppler (PW), continuous wave Doppler (CW), colour Doppler, three-dimensional (3-D), tissue Doppler (TDI). This chapter will focus on 2-D, and mention M-mode and Doppler modes.

▷ Two-dimensional echocardiography

Two-dimensional echocardiography demonstrates the spatial relationship of structures and therefore provides an accurate anatomical diagnosis of abnormalities in the heart and great vessels. It provides tomographic images of the heart by directing the transducer beam along selected cross-sectional planes.

Once this skill is mastered with a clear understanding of the normal sequential anatomy, abnormalities in anatomy or function can be diagnosed at least to start emergency management until a more experienced echocardiographer is available.

The standard imaging planes are shown in Figure 1.

Sequential analysis during 2-D echocardiography

The following sequence is often performed to ensure a complete, systematic approach:

1. Abdominal situs
2. Atrio-ventricular concordance
3. Ventriculo-arterial concordance
4. Shunts: atrial septal defect (ASD), ventricular septal defect (VSD), patent ductus arteriosus (PDA)
5. Aortic arch, head and neck vessels, and descending aorta
6. Pulmonary venous drainage
7. Systemic venous drainage
8. Global function
9. Pericardial collection

ECHOCARDIOGRAPHY

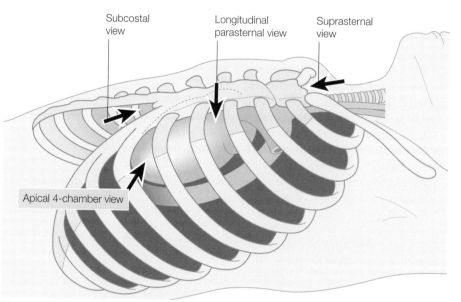

Figure 1 Imaging sequence and planes.

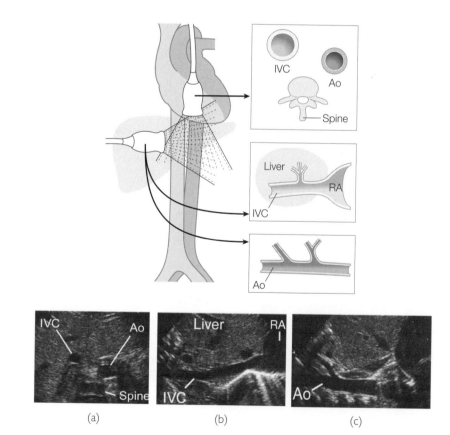

Figure 2 Abdominal transverse (a) and parasagittal (b, c) views. IVC, inferior vena cava; RA, right atrium; Ao, aorta.

ECHOCARDIOGRAPHY

In paediatric cardiology we use the above standard sequence and additional views may be varied as follows.

Abdominal parasagittal and transverse views (Figure 2)

In paediatrics we start with the abdominal transverse view to determine the situs and pulsation of the abdominal aorta. These are obtained from the subxiphoid region, and are useful to demonstrate the inferior vena cava (IVC), hepatic veins (HV) and abdominal aorta (Abd Ao).

- The transverse abdominal plane (Figure 2a) shows the liver on the right side and the stomach on the left, cross-section of the spine is seen posteriorly with the aorta (Ao) left and posterior and the IVC right and anterior.
- In the sagittal plane (Figure 2b), slight rightward angulation of the transducer demonstrates the IVC passing through the liver and entering the right atrium (RA); minor angulation will demonstrate the hepatic vein joining the IVC just below the RA.
- Leftward angulation provides a longitudinal view of the abdominal aorta; often the coeliac and superior mesenteric arteries can be visualised from the anterior wall of the aorta (Figure 2c).

Subcostal views (Figure 3)

Subcostal views are perpendicular to the four-chamber views; the transducer is in the subxiphoid region and is rotated about 90 degrees clockwise from the four-chamber view and is visualised as if looking from the patient's left side.

- The most rightward plane (Figure 3a) transects the superior (SVC) and inferior vena cavae and their connection to the right atrium.
- Leftward angulation passes the ultrasound beam through the body of the right ventricle (RV) and outflow tract to the pulmonary valve (PV) (Figure 3b).
- More angulation to the left provides short axis view of the left ventricle (LV) and papillary muscles (PM) and the mitral valve (MV) (Figure 3b, c).

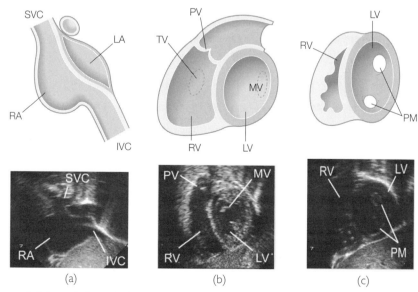

Figure 3 Subcostal views. SVC, superior vena cava; IVC, inferior vena cava; RA, right atrium; LA, left atrium; PV, pulmonary vein; TV, tricuspid valve; MV, mitral valve; RV, right ventricle; LV, left ventricle; PM, papillary muscles.

Additional subcostal views: angulated sagittal views (Figure 4)

- Section a: More posterior angulation shows the coronary sinus (CS), left and right atriums (RA, LA) and pulmonary veins draining to the LA;
- Section b: Less posterior tilt: descending thoracic aorta (DAo), pulmonary veins to LA;
- Section c: Anterior tilt: superior vena cava (SVC) to RA, LV to aorta;
- Section d: More anterior tilt: inlet/outlet view of the right ventricle right atrium to right ventricle through the tricuspid valve (TV), then the right ventricular outflow tract (RVOT) to pulmonary artery (PA) through the pulmonary valve, and branch pulmonary arteries more distally.

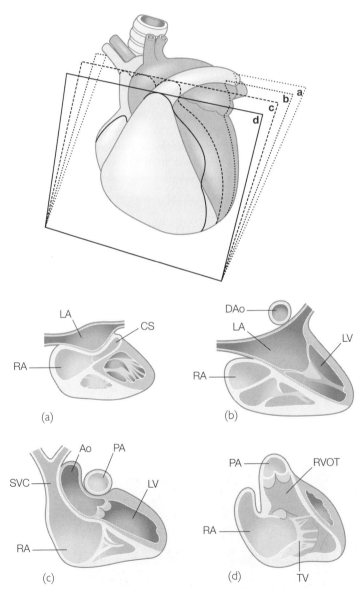

Figure 4 Angulated sagittal view. SVC, superior vena cava; RA, right atrium; LA, left atrium; TV, tricuspid valve; RV, right ventricle; LV, left ventricle; CS, coronary sinus; Ao, aorta; PA, pulmonary artery; DAo, descending thoracic aorta; RVOT, right ventricular outflow tract.

Four-chamber views (Figure 5)

Four-chamber views are obtained by placing the transducer on the cardiac apex. From there, angulation anterior and posterior will give three standard imaging planes.

- Anterior angulation provides the five-chamber (outlet) view: the four chambers plus the aortic valve, subaortic area, proximal part of the ascending aorta, sometimes the left coronary artery, and outlet part of the interventricular septum (IVS) (Figure 5a). Some echocardiographers can visualise the pulmonary artery arising from the right ventricle by further anterior angulation of the transducer, but this is not a standard view.
- Anterior tilting demonstrates the standard four-chamber (inlet) view, in which the four cardiac chambers are seen: two atria and two balanced ventricles; the two AV valves, tricuspid (TV) and mitral (MV) with normal offsetting, the inlet part of interventricular septum (IVS) and the pulmonary veins (Figure 5b).
- Posterior angulation provides the coronary sinus (CS) view, RA and tricuspid valve (Figure 5c).

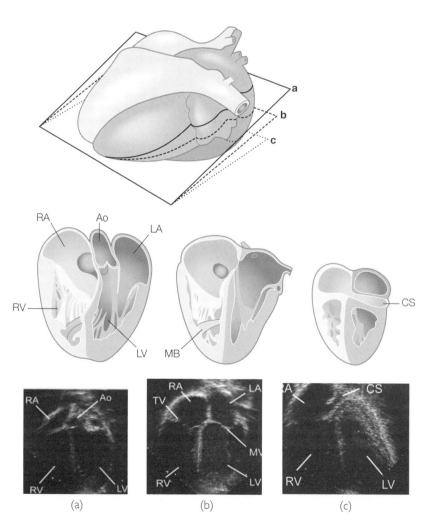

Figure 5 Four-chamber views.

Left parasternal long axis view (Figure 6)

The transducer is placed in the third or fourth intercostal spaces angulating at the 11 o'clock position with the aorta to the right. The left ventricular cavity is to the left of the screen with both mitral and aortic valves clearly seen, the left ventricular cavity is not foreshortened, and the left atrium is behind the ascending aorta and the right ventricular cavity, and the outflow tract is most anterior at 12 o'clock position.

- Motion of the aortic and mitral valve leaflets is apparent.
- Normal continuity of the anterior mitral valve leaflet with the posterior aortic root.
- M-mode analysis of LV function and dimensions and aortic to LA ratio can be done from this view.

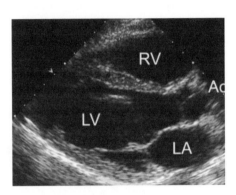

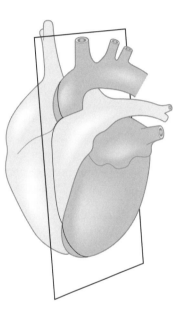

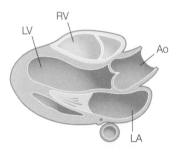

Figure 6 Left parasternal lung axis view.

Left parasternal short axis views (Figure 7)

With the transducer in the same third or fourth intercostal spaces where optimum long axis view was obtained, rotate the transducer by 90 degrees. The images are shown as if looking superiorly from the apex of the heart.

- Most superior plane: the aortic valve is seen in cross-section in the middle of the screen with its typical three cusps, the right ventricular outflow tract anteriorly leading to the pulmonary valve to the left of the aortic valve and the main pulmonary artery in the longitudinal plane giving rise to the right and left branch pulmonary arteries. The tricuspid valve is to the right and the interatrial septum is at the 7 o'clock position separating the right and left atriums. Ductal flow may be demonstrated here but a higher cut towards the aortic arch is better. Coronary arteries can be easily visualised in this section bearing in mind that the right coronary artery arises at a higher level than the left (Figure 7a).
- The mid-level plane transects the left ventricle and the mitral valve, which has a characteristic fish-mouth appearance surrounded by the left ventricular endocardium. This is a good position to assess wall motion abnormalities, M-mode analysis and mitral valve abnormalities (Figure 7b).
- Inferior plane: there is further inferior angulation. Medial angulation from the papillary muscles of the left ventricle permits visualisation of the anterior and/or septal leaflets of the tricuspid valve (Figure 7c).

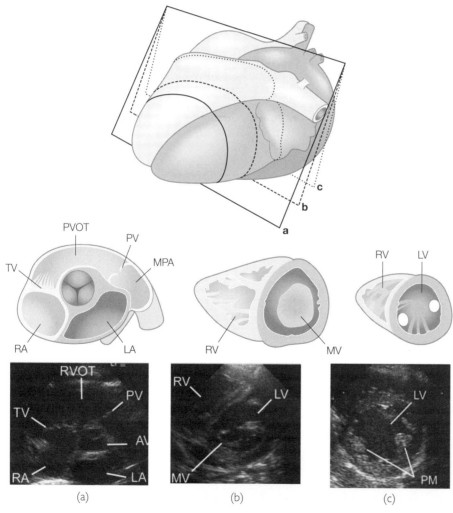

Figure 7 Left parasternal short axis views.

ECHOCARDIOGRAPHY

Suprasternal views (Figure 8)

In neonates and infants the suprasternal view is better obtained just to the right of the suprasternal notch in the right first intercostal space angulating the transducer to the left between the 5 o'clock and 7 o'clock positions.

- Long axis (arch) view: illustrates the ascending aorta (AAo), aortic arch, isthmus and descending aorta (DAo). The innominate vein may be visualised anterior to the arch and traced to the right superior vena cava. The origin of the three head and neck vessels (innominate artery (IA) and left common carotid and subclavian arteries) is seen (Figure 8a). The arterial duct can be easily seen as well.
- Transverse view (three-vessel view): aortic arch in cross-section with the SVC to the right and the pulmonary artery posterior and to the left giving rise to the right pulmonary artery (RPA). In the posterior part of the image, the LA can be demonstrated with the four pulmonary veins (PV) (Figure 8b). With angulation to the left a better profile of the ductus can be obtained.

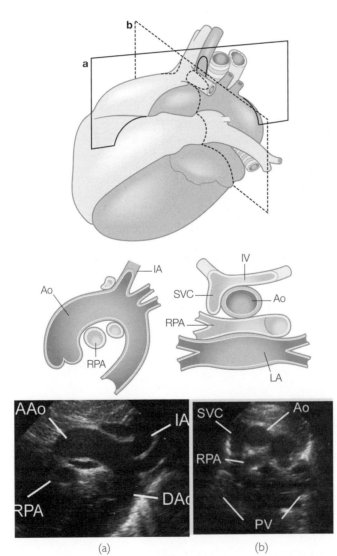

Figure 8 Suprasternal views.

▷ M-mode

This modality, which is created by a very narrow ultrasound beam plotted against time, is important in evaluation of cardiac function, measurement of dimensions and timing. It is used for:

- Measurement of cardiac dimensions and wall thickness (Figure 9)
- LV systolic function:
  - Fractional shortening: normal value 28–44%
  - Ejection fraction: normal value 64–83%
- Assessment of valve motion
- Detection of pericardial fluid

Normal M-mode echo measurements are given in Table 1.

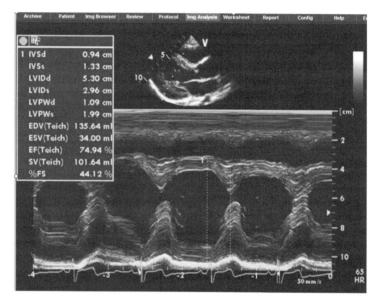

Figure 9 M-mode in parasternal view. Note: (i) the aortic valve and mitral valves have to be clearly open and (ii) the interventricular septum and posterior left ventricular walls have to be parallel and the sector taken at exactly 90 degrees through the tip of the mitral valve.

▷ Doppler-based modes

Colour flow mapping

This is colour-coded Doppler superimposed on the 2-D image demonstrating the direction and turbulence in the blood flow across cardiac structures. The coding is red towards the transducer, blue away from the transducer, and a mosaic of red, blue and yellow in turbulent flow. Shunt and regurgitant valve leaks can be seen and evaluated.

Doppler echocardiography

Doppler echocardiography detects frequency shifts which enable the detection of blood flow velocity and direction. The pulsed Doppler provides precise sampling site but the maximum velocity is limited so at high velocities aliasing becomes a limiting factor. Then, continuous Doppler (CW) has to be used instead.

ECHOCARDIOGRAPHY

Table 1 Normal M-mode echo measurements (mm): mean (95 per cent prediction interval)

BW (kg)	3	5	8	10	15	20	25	30	40	50	60	70
BSA (m²)	0.24	0.34	0.45	0.52	0.68	0.82	0.94	1.06	1.27	1.47	1.65	1.82
IVS	4.5 (3.5–5)	4.5 (4–5.5)	5 (4.5–6)	5.5 (4.5–6)	6 (5–7)	7 (5.5–8.5)	7 (5.5–9)	7.5 (6–9)	8.5 (6.5–10)	8.5 (7–10)	9 (8–10.5)	9.5 (7.5–11)
LVPW	4 (3.5–5)	4.5 (4–5)	5 (4–6)	5 (4.5–6)	6 (5–7)	6.5 (5.5–8)	7 (6–8)	7 (6–8.5)	8 (6.5–9)	8.5 (7–9.5)	8.5 (7.5–10)	9 (7.5–11)
AO	12 (10–14)	13 (11–16)	15 12–17	16 (13–18)	18 (15–22)	19 16–23	21 (17–24)	22 (18–26)	23 (19–27)	25 (20–29)	26 21–30	27 (23–32)
LA	18 (15–21)	20 (16–23)	21 (17–25)	22 (18–26)	25 (21–29)	27 (22–32)	28 (23–33)	30 (24–35)	32 (26–37)	34 (28–41)	36 (29–42)	
LVDD	21 (18–23)	25 (22–27)	28 (24–31)	29 (25–32)	33 (29–36)	35 (31–39)	37 (33–41)	39 (34–43)	42 (37–47)	44 (39–49)	46 (41–51)	48 (42–53)
LVSD	14 (12–17)	16 (13–19)	17 (14–21)	18 (15–22)	21 (17–24)	23 (18–27)	24 (19–28)	24 (21–29)	27 (22–32)	28 (23–33)	29 (24–34)	31 (25–36)

Adapted from Ware H et al. Circulation 1987;57:278–87. Although it is an old publication, it still holds up as the newer ones tended to underestimate the measurements.

AO, ascending aorta; BSA, body surface area; BW, body weight; IVS, interventricular septum; LA, left atrium; LVDD, left ventricular diastolic dimension; LVPW, left ventricular posterior wall; LVSD, left ventricular systolic dimension.

Using the Bernoulli equation, the pressure gradient across a restriction (e.g. pulmonary valve) can be derived indirectly. Regurgitant flow across the tricuspid valve in the presence of pulmonary hypertension provides an indirect means of estimating the RV (and hence the pulmonary artery) systolic blood pressure.

▷ Interpretation of abnormalities

Diagnosing a major abnormality which has been missed during general fetal screening, and which is duct dependent, can be life-saving. The first to be faced with this problem is often the neonatologist or paediatrician, presented with a collapsed newborn baby in the emergency department. Examples of this situation include:

- Duct-dependent pulmonary circulation: critical pulmonary stenosis, pulmonary atresia, tricuspid atresia
- Duct-dependent systemic circulation: critical aortic stenosis, coarctation, interruption aortic arch, hypoplastic left heart syndrome
- Cyanotic non-duct-dependent: obstructed total anomalous pulmonary venous drainage (TAPVD), Fallot's tetralogy
- Lesions presenting with high cardiac output heart failure and (if prolonged) pulmonary hypertension: truncus, complete atrio-ventricular septal defect (CAVSD), large left to right shunt.

▷ Further reading

Snider RA. *Echocardiography in Paediatric Heart Disease*, 2nd edn. Edinburgh: Mosby, 1997.
Gera R. *Step by Step Paediatric Echocardiography*. London: Taylor & Francis, 2004.
Everett AD, Scott LD. *Illustrated Field Guide to Congenital Heart Disease and Repair*. Scientific Software Solutions, 2005.

ECHOCARDIOGRAPHY

▶ Background and indications

The electrocardiogram (ECG) provides much useful clinical information about the function and rhythm of the heart, even in the era of advanced cardiac imaging. It is used in the assessment of every cardiac patient and in paediatric practice on suspicion of a cardiac, structural, rhythm or conduction problem. The interpretation rarely provides a specific diagnosis. The ECG may also be valuable in assessing the impact of electrolyte disturbances.

▷ The standard ECG

Electrode positions (Figure 1)

- Standard (I, II, III) and unipolar leads (aVR, aVF, aVL) same as adults
- Precordial leads V1–V6, with V4R, V3R
- In dextrocardia V6R to V1
- A rhythm strip with three leads or lead II to assess rhythm disturbances

Recording

- Speed 25 mm/s (1 small square = 0.04 s)
- At full standardisation amplitude of 10 mm = 1 mV
- Recording at 50 mm/s helps in interval measurement where extra precision is needed

The standard deflections and the intervals which may be measured are illustrated in Figure 2.

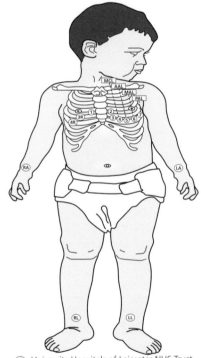

© University Hospitals of Leicester NHS Trust

Figure 1 Electrode positions for standard ECG. Redrawn with permission from University Hospitals of Leicester NHS Trust.

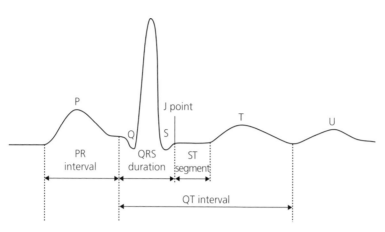

Figure 2 Deflections and intervals.

Pitfalls

- The main sources of artefact are excessive motion and poor electrical contact. These should be detected and corrected during recording.
- Significant changes in the form (quality) and the amplitudes and intervals (quantity) occur during development and should be taken into account by referral to age-related standards.

▷ Interpretation

First make sure the ECG corresponds to the patient in question with date and date of birth.

Order of ECG interpretation

1. Rate and rhythm
2. AV conduction (PR interval)
3. Atrial de/repolarisation (P wave)
4. Ventricular depolarisation (QRS)
5. Ventricular repolarisation (T wave)
6. Hypertrophy, enlargement

Rate and rhythm

■ Heart rate

Heart rate (HR) is influenced by body temperature, autonomic nervous system (anxiety), activity and age. It is determined from the ECG by: HR = 300/No. of large (0.2) squares or 1500/No. of small (0.04) squares in the R-R interval. Normal age variations should be appreciated:

- Premature and low birthweight infants: 77–211 bpm.
- Full-term neonate: minimum 55–75 to 220 bpm; 3–33 per cent of neonates have atrial (APC) or ventricular premature contractions (VPC).
- Older children: minimum 44–68, maximum 132–196 bpm; 15–40 per cent have APCs, and VPCs occur in 3 per cent as non-sustained ventricular tachycardia.
- Fit adolescents especially athletes: 31–55 bpm, causing some monitoring equipment to alarm.
- Sinus pauses <3 s, 1st degree and 2nd degree (type 1) heart block can be normal variations.

ELECTROCARDIOGRAPHY

▪ Rhythm

Rhythms should be defined as regular, irregular or regular with intermittent predictable irregularity. The relationship of P waves to the QRS complexes defines the rhythm.

Sinus P wave represents atrial depolarisation from top to bottom and from right to left and is thus positive in I, II, aVF and negative in aVR. Reversal of P wave vector occurs in situs inversus.

AV conduction

- First degree heart block is prolonged PR interval without dropped beats.
- Second degree heart block leads to lost beats, either type 1 progressive increase in PR interval until beat dropped (Wenckebach's phenomenon) or type 2 intermittent dropped beats without lengthened PR interval.
- Third degree heart block is complete heart block, i.e. no relation between P and QRS complexes.

Atrial depolarisation

The P wave initially involves the right atrium and later left atrial components. Its duration:

- Infancy: 0.04–0.07s
- Adolescence: 0.06–0.1s

It is tallest in leads II, V4R, V1 (upper limit 2.5 mm). Variable pattern implies an anomalous pacemaker.

Atrial hypertrophy is recognised as follows:

- Right atrial hypertrophy: spiked P wave >2.5 mm in II, V4R, V1, occurring in severe pulmonary or tricuspid obstructions or in pulmonary hypertension.
- Left atrial hypertrophy: notched P wave or large negative component in V4R, V1, indicating mitral valve disease, LV cardiomyopathy.

Ventricular depolarisation

The *QRS complex* varies a little with age. Its duration is:

- 0–8 years: <80 ms (2 small squares)
- Over 8 years: <90 ms

The duration is prolonged in:

- R or L bundle branch block
- Ventricular pre-excitation
- Ventricular pace-maker
- Ventricular hypertrophy
- Intraventricular conduction delay: CMP, ARVD.

The *Q wave* represents depolarisation of the interventricular septum from L to R and is seen in leads II, III, aVF, V5 and V6; it measures 2–3 mm (>4 mm is abnormal) and its duration is <40 ms. There are prominent Q waves in left ventricular hypertrophy and biventricular hypertrophy. Q waves in other leads are rare and are seen in hypertrophic obstructive cardiomyopathy, absent left coronary artery syndrome and complete congenital transposition of the great arteries. R and S sizes are determined by ventricular wall thickness, which varies with age.

QRS axis is the direction of maximal electrical force during depolarisation (Figure 3).

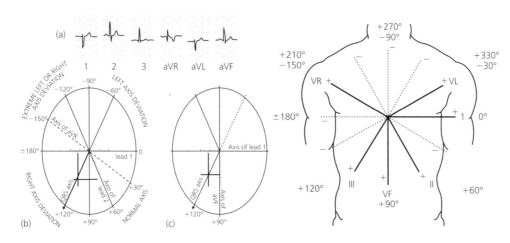

Figure 3 Calculation of QRS axis.

- Method 1: using leads I and II, plot amplitudes of R-S in leads I and II; drop perpendiculars from those axes; line from origin through intersection is the electrical axis.
- Method 2: using leads I and aVF, repeat method 1, enhancing amplitude of AVF by 1.3.
- Method 3: choose any limb lead with R=S; electrical axis will be at right angles to the axis of that lead.

Ventricular repolarisation

ST-T wave abnormalities are defined as: elevation >0.1 mV or depression ≤0.05 mV; affected by electrolyte disturbance, myocarditis, pericarditis, infarction or drugs.

QT interval is HR and age dependent; QTc=QT /√previous RR in lead II and has values of:

- 0–6 months <0.490 s
- >6 months <0.425 s

Increased Q occurs in certain familial syndromes and with electrolytes and metabolic disturbance and some drugs.

T wave should measure a quarter to a third of the R wave; upright in V4R, V1±V2, V3 then inverted after third day of life; remains inverted in Rt chest leads until early adolescence, then becomes upright in V2, V3 (5–15 years); normally inverted in aVR, ± aVF, III; T wave is always inverted in V1 unless there is a pathology; inverted T in other leads due to ventricular hypertrophy, myocardial disease, pericarditis and severe hypothyroidism.

Ventricular hypertrophy

■ Criteria for left ventricular hypertrophy

1. Mild LVH: sum of S in V1+R in V5 or V6 >30 mm under 1 year or >40 mm over 1 year
2. Moderate LVH: 1 + prolonged QRS or flat T wave in V5, V6
3. Severe LVH: 1 + 2 + T wave inversion in V5, V6

■ **Causes**
- Aortic valve disease
- Moderate size ventricular septal defect
- Large patent ductus arteriosus
- Mitral regurgitation
- Systemic hypertension
- Congestive and obstructive cardiomyopathy

■ **Criteria for right ventricular hypertrophy**
1. Mild RVH: right axis deviation, R wave above normal limits in V4R, V1 R>S in V1 after age of 12 months; S wave in V6 greater than normal of age: 15 mm in first week, 10 mm 1–24 week, 7 mm 6–12 months, 5 mm >1 year
2. Moderate RVH: 1 + prolonged QRS and upright T wave in V4R, V1 after 3 days of age
3. Severe RVH: tall R waves in V4R, V1 QRS >90 ms and deep T wave inversion in V4R, V1

■ **Causes**
- Pulmonary stenosis
- Pulmonary hypertension
- Fallot tetralogy
- Right bundle branch block
- Wolff–Parkinson–White syndrome

■ **Biventricular hypertrophy**
Biventricular hypertrophy is detected by: tall R and deep S in V3, V4 (R+S >50 mm at any age); LVH + wide or bifid R in V4R, V1 >8 mm; RVH + T wave inversion V5–6 (T upright in V1–2) or Q wave ≥3 mm in V5–6; criteria of RVH, LVH.

▷ **ECG examples**

(a) Complete AVSD: note superior axis (+90 degrees)

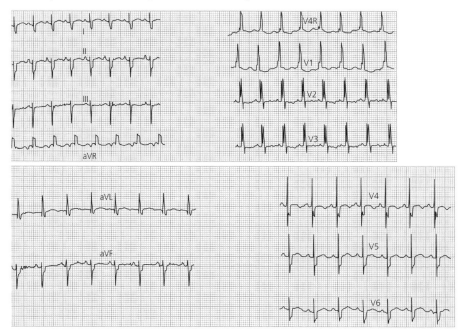

(b) Partial right bundle block PRBBB, normal heart

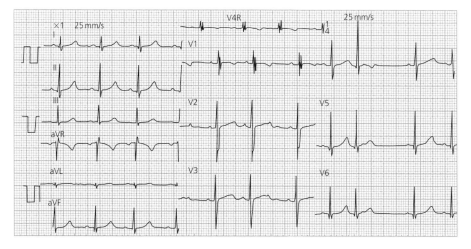

Figure 4 ECG examples.

ELECTROCARDIOGRAPHY

(c) Complete right bundle block: post-VSD closure

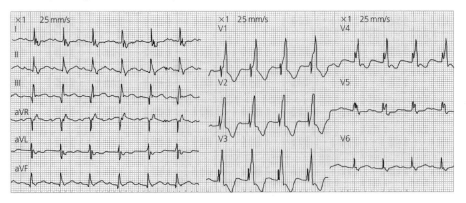

(d) Hypoplastic left heart syndrome: decreased LV forces not RVH

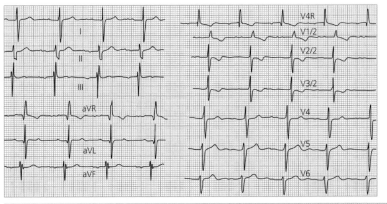

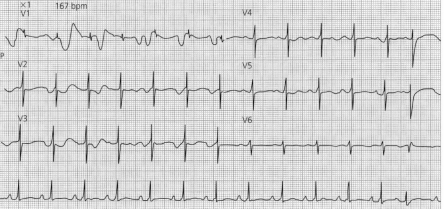

Figure 4 *(continued)*

(e) Tricuspid atresia: decreased RV forces not LVH

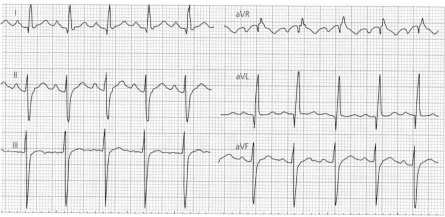

(f) Congenitally corrected TGA: Q in V4R and V1

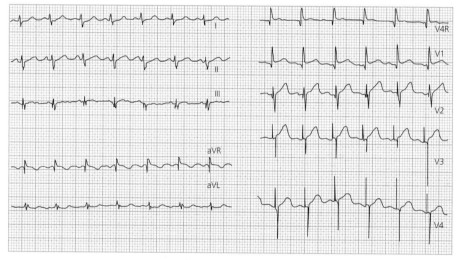

Figure 4 *(continued)*

ELECTROCARDIOGRAPHY

(g) Anomalous left coronary artery from pulmonary artery: notice deep Q waves

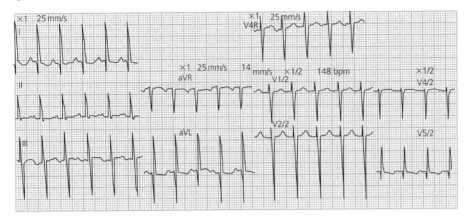

(h) Dilated cardiomyopathy: note T wave inversion in V5–6

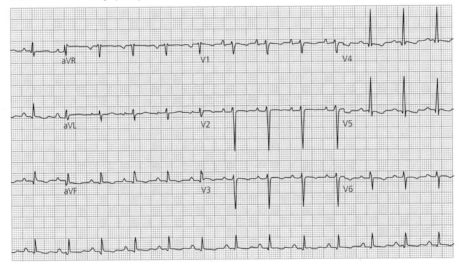

Figure 4 *(continued)*

(i) Atrial ectopics

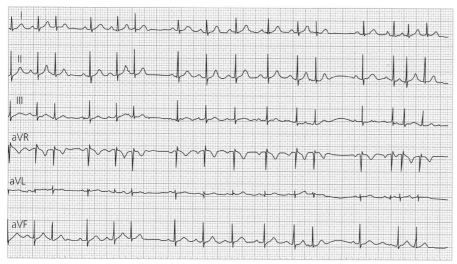

(j) Ventricular ectopics

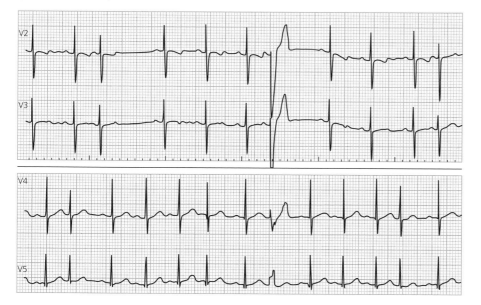

Figure 4 *(continued)*

(k) Complete heart block

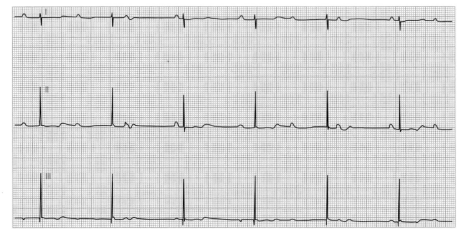

Figure 4 *(continued)*

▷ Further reading

Park MK, Guneroth WG. *How to Read Pediatric ECGs.* Edinburgh: Mosby Elsevier, 2006.

► Indications

The aim of the nasogastric tube is to:

- Allow drainage of stomach contents
- Allow removal of air from the stomach especially in ventilated patients and those on continuous positive airway pressure (CPAP)
- Provide an access route to the gastrointestinal tract for the safe administration of fluids, drugs and nutrients

▷ Contraindications/cautions for nasogastric tube insertion

- Maxillofacial disorders, particularly following trauma
- Confirmed or suspected base of skull fractures
- Established clotting problems/disorders
- Infants with nasal obstruction
- Infants in severe respiratory distress

▷ Types of nasogastic tube

Two types of nasogastric tube are available for infants and children:

- Polyvinyl chloride tubes for short-term use (up to 10 days)
- Polyurethane tubes for long-term use (>10 days)

▷ Procedure

Equipment

- Nasogastric tube of appropriate size
- Hypoallergenic tape
- pH paper
- Working suction and syringe to aspirate the tube

Position

Infants under the age of 1 year might be better managed wrapped securely in a blanket as long as it is possible to observe their colour and chest movement. Older children can have the tube inserted while in the upright position if they are not mechanically ventilated.

Method

1. Select the appropriate length of the tube by measuring the distance from child's ear lobe to the tip of the nose to the xiphisternum.
2. Lubricate the tube with sterile warm water and insert the tube into the clearest nostril and slide it backwards and inwards along the floor of the nasopharynx. If there is any obstruction try again in a slightly different direction or use the other nostril.
3. Pass the tube to the predetermined mark and secure it along the side of the face with hypoallergenic tape.

In a cooperative older child a swallowing action closes the glottis and enables the tube to pass into the oesophagus.

NASOGASTRIC TUBE INSERTION

Helpful hints

- If the patient shows signs of respiratory distress, the tube should be withdrawn immediately. Should the tube meet resistance/cannot be advanced, the practitioner should not make more than three attempts to insert the tube and should seek help. Confirm correct placement before feeding the child.
- Do not use litmus paper to confirm the position of the tube but use pH paper. pH paper test strips detect a 0.5 pH increment. pH measurements of below 5 indicate that the tube is correctly positioned and can be used.
- Ensure the tube that you place is of an adequate size as a small tube will be suboptimal in draining fluid and air from the stomach.
- The position of the tube must not be confirmed by auscultation as this method is unsafe and unreliable.

▶ Background

Gastro-oesophageal reflux (GOR) is defined as the passive transfer of gastric contents into the oesophagus. Several factors may be involved including transient or chronic relaxation of the lower oesophageal sphincter, oesophageal dysmotility and delayed gastric emptying. It is a normal phenomenon in infants, reducing in frequency with age.

Gastro-oesophageal reflux disease (GORD) is defined as GOR causing symptoms or complications. GORD may need further investigation and management.

A good history and examination is sufficient to distinguish between simple reflux (GOR) needing only reassurance and advice, and GORD and warning symptoms or signs that necessitate further management.

Initial management of GORD may include advice regarding feed frequency, volumes positioning and timing. A trial of 2 weeks of milk-free diet may be appropriate in a young infant, especially if there is eczema or a family history of atopy. After this a trial of antireflux medication should be reserved for those infants in whom GORD persists, together with complications (see Table 1).

Table 1 Symptoms and complications of gastro-oesophageal reflux disease

Gastrointestinal symptoms/complications	Extra-gastrointestinal symptoms/complications
Pain, heartburn (older child)	Wheeze
Feed-related crying and distress (infant)	Recurrent aspiration
Failure to thrive	Pneumonia (especially in neurologically impaired)
Haematemesis	Apparent life-threatening events
Anaemia	Apnoea (neonatal apnoea is not usually due to gastro-oesophageal reflux)
Oesophagitis	
Barrett's oesophagus (rare in children)	

Only in cases where symptoms persist despite the above measures should further investigation, such as 24-hour pH monitoring, be considered. More recent research suggests that combined pH and multichannel oesophageal impedance monitoring may in the future become the investigation of choice, but at present this is not routinely available.

▷ Indications

pH monitoring should only be used as above if there is GORD unresponsive to simple measures and antireflux medication, rather than just simple GOR.

Investigation of possible GORD may include a barium meal and follow through (to delineate anatomy, oesophagogastroduodenoscopy (OGD) and biopsy for the histological picture and exclude other diagnoses such as eosinophilic oesophagitis), as well as the 24-hour oesophageal pH monitoring.

pH monitoring is also used if respiratory symptoms such as chronic wheeze, or even ENT symptoms such as chronic rhinitis, fail to respond to appropriate therapy and reflux is suspected.

▷ Contraindications

pH monitoring cannot be done if feeds are more frequent than 3 hourly as acid stomach contents will be buffered and reflux events missed.

▷ Equipment

A pH probe is inserted to 5 cm above the lower oesophageal sphincter (if manometry is used) or to the level of the third vertebra above the diaphragm on X-ray. These probes are disposable and come in different sizes depending on age.

The test gives a 24-hour continuous reading of pH in the lower (and sometimes upper) oesophagus. The 24-hour printout is downloaded onto a computer with appropriate software at the end of the study. Recordings are stored and can be read or reviewed at a later time.

▷ Consideration of the different age groups

There are challenges in passing the probe in younger children due to discomfort (see below).

Clearly interpretation depends on age (see below) with higher levels of reflux acceptable as normal in infants under 1 year.

Pitfalls

- Insertion of the probe is very similar to nasogastric tube insertion and as such can be uncomfortable. While a young infant can be wrapped up and cuddled to aid insertion, an older child must cooperate, and hence insertion can sometimes fail. In children in whom oesophagogastroduodenoscopy (OGD) is also being done, insertion under general anaesthesia will help reduce these problems.
- Care must be taken before starting the recording that the probe is correctly positioned. In adults manometry can help, but this technique is difficult in children and hence is not used. Fluoroscopy can show tip position and ensure no curling of the tube, but in practice, X-ray is the most common tool for checking the position. There are formulae available to predict oesophageal length (OL) (such as Strobel's – OL from nares to lower oesophageal sphincter = (height in cm × 0.252) + 5). The probe is inserted to 87 per cent of this length, but X-ray conformation is still needed.
- Interpretation (see below) can be difficult, and it needs to be remembered that the probe only picks up *acid* reflux – alkaline reflux will be missed. This is the potential advantage with intra-oesophageal electrical impedance monitoring which picks up *all* reflux, but normal ranges for impedance monitoring have yet to be determined.

▷ Results and their interpretation

The results come as a printout of pH values over 24 hours, and a table of the number and timing of reflux events, along with the Reflux Index (see Table 2). This is the percentage of the time that the pH is below 4. In interpreting these, a reflux event has been deemed to take place if pH goes below 4 for at least 15 seconds.

Table 2 Normal values for the Reflux Index

Age	Normal Reflux Index
Under 1	Up to 10%
Over 1	Up to 5%

As above, reflux is a normal phenomenon, especially in infants and also in older children and adults. There are some normal ranges available but these are based on fairly small numbers.

Parameters used in interpreting a pH recording
- Percentage of time pH is under 4 (Reflux Index)
- Number of reflux episodes and number of prolonged episodes (>5 minutes)
- Duration of longest reflux episode
- A record of events (e.g. meals, sleep, respiratory symptoms) to determine whether reflux events coincide with symptoms

Using these parameters, judgement can be made of the severity of the GORD, or whether the symptoms shown are indeed due to the GORD.

▷ Further reading

Rudolph C, Mazur LJ, Liptak GS, *et al.* Guidelines for the evaluation and treatment of gastro-oesophageal reflux in infants and children: recommendations of the North American Society for pediatrics. *J Paediatr Gastroenterol Nutr* 2001;**32**(Suppl. 2):S1–31.

INSERTION OF OESOPHAGEAL pH PROBE

COLONOSCOPY

▶ **Background**

The procedure of colonoscopy should more correctly be referred to as ileocolonoscopy, as in children a full examination including terminal ileum should be the aim, even if this is not always technically possible. As with oesophagogastroduodenoscopy, ileocolonoscopy has been central to diagnosis and treatment of a number of gastrointestinal conditions since the 1970s. Currently video endoscopes are used. The picture is seen on a connected video unit, which means that observers can see the pictures as well as the endoscopist.

▷ **Indications**

- Diagnosis of suspected inflammatory bowel disease
- Investigation of chronic diarrhoea or per rectum blood loss
- Surveillance of known inflammatory bowel disease (IBD), especially if resistant to first line treatment
- Suspected colitis due to other causes, e.g. allergic colitis, or rarer causes

▷ **Procedure**

In adults ileocolonoscopy is performed under sedation, but in children the procedure is normally performed under general anaesthesia. Older teenagers can sometimes tolerate the procedure under sedation.

All children having ileocolonoscopy need bowel preparation with clear fluids only for 24 hours prior to the procedure, and laxative administration (such as Picolax, or a combination of sodium picosulphate and senna in one or two high doses) to clear the bowel. A rectal washout 1 hour before can help, especially if the faecal fluid is not clear. Diagnostic ileocolonoscopy involves passing a flexible endoscope via the anus round the large bowel as far as the caecum, and on through the ileocaecal valve into the terminal ileum.

Therapeutic ileocolonoscopy additionally mainly involves removal of polyps, with other procedures such as dilation of strictures rarely performed in children.

▷ **Equipment**

A detailed description of all the different endoscopes is outside the remit of this book, but they do come in different diameters to suit the size of patient. They all have an instrument channel, and accessory channels to insufflate air or inject or aspirate water. To perform colonoscopy, the following are essential:

- an endoscopy suite or suitably equipped theatre
- staff trained to assist in endoscopy, including the cleaning and disinfecting of scopes
- an anaesthetist and an operating department practitioner – if procedures are done under general anaesthesia
- sufficient endoscopes to run a list (the cleaning process takes over 30 minutes)
- a suitably trained endoscopist

It is possible (see below) to perform colonoscopy in older teenagers under sedation, in which case an anaesthetist or paediatrician trained to give sedation safely and effectively is needed as well as the endoscopist and paediatric trained nursing staff.

Consideration of different age groups

The size of scope depends on the size of the child. As stated above, it is possible to perform colonoscopy on older teenagers under sedation. This is sometimes not ideal, but if suitably trained staff give the sedation, and the teenager and family are given information about both options it can work well.

Pitfalls

- A number of specific problems may occur, as well as the general complications of procedure under anaesthetic.
- Perforation or bleeding may occur.
- Poor quality biopsy samples may limit interpretation. In patchy colitis it is important to take a biopsy sample of normal as well as abnormal mucosa, in order to demonstrate the patchy nature of the disease.

▷ Results and their interpretation

Results from ileocolonoscopy consist of:

- macroscopic findings – a description is written, photos can be taken and the video can also be recorded and kept for future reference
- histological findings – always required in addition, and give more detailed information

Some of the commonest diagnoses are given below along with the macroscopic and microscopic findings.

Crohn's disease

Crohn's disease produces changes that are patchy not just macroscopically but microscopically, with variable inflammation within a single biopsy. The diagnostic feature of Crohn's disease is granulomas (only present in 30–40 per cent, and may be present in, for example, tuberculosis). They need to be distinguished from microgranuloma or a histolytic reaction associated with a disrupted crypt, which is not a specific finding for Crohn's disease. More severe Crohn's disease may produce cobblestoning, which results from linear ulceration with oedematous mucosa in between.

Changes present in the ileum are usually diagnostic of Crohn's disease (although backwash ileitis may be present in ulcerative colitis – see below). Inflammation is transmural, although this would not be picked up in mucosal endoscopic biopsies.

Ulcerative colitis

As a rule, in ulcerative colitis abnormalities are found in the rectum and spread proximally. The extent varies but it rarely goes beyond the ileocaecal valve, although in pancolitis there is sometimes backwash ileitis.

Ulcers may be seen (from small through to larger 'geographical' ulcers). There is more uniform inflammation with abnormal distorted shortened or branched crypts much more obvious than in Crohn's. Lesions are limited to the mucosa, although as above this would not be picked up in endoscopic biopsies.

Indeterminate colitis

A small percentage of patients with IBD have indeterminate colitis. There are macroscopic and microscopic features of definite IBD, but without diagnostic feature of either Crohn's disease or ulcerative colitis.

COLONOSCOPY

Practical Paediatric Procedures

▷ **Further reading**

Gershman G, Ament M (eds). *Practical Pediatric Gastrointestinal Endoscopy*. Oxford: Wiley-Blackwell Publishing, 2007.

Walker WA, Goulet O, Kleinman RA, *et al.* (eds). *Pediatric Gastrointestinal Disease*. Philadelphia: BC Decker Inc, 2004.

OESOPHAGOGASTRODUODENOSCOPY

▶ Background

Oesophagogastroduodenoscopy (OGD) has become a primary investigation for a number of conditions since the first paediatric endoscope was developed in the 1970s. Early fibreoptic endoscopes with a view only for the endoscopist have been replaced by video endoscopes where the picture is seen on a connected video unit.

Diagnostic endoscopy involves passing a flexible tube down the oesophagus as far as the duodenum/jejunum under general anaesthesia, in order to visualise the upper gastrointestinal tract and take biopsies. Therapeutic endoscopy additionally involves performing other procedures such as dilatation of strictures or banding of oesophageal varices. In the UK, guidelines as to who should undertake OGD (and ileocolonoscopy) in children have recently been published by the British Society of Paediatric Gastroenterology Hepatology and Nutrition (BSPGHAN). Only those who have sufficient experience and a competence-based assessment should attempt this procedure.

Indications

Indications for OGD in children are shown in Table 1, but the whole clinical picture must be taken into account in making a decision about whether OGD is needed. The indications and diagnoses vary with age.

- To confirm coeliac disease: although modern coeliac screens including TTG (tissue transglutaminase) have a very high sensitivity and specificity, duodenal biopsy (×4) is still recommended to confirm the diagnosis prior to treatment.
- To investigate possible inflammatory bowel disease (IBD): OGD and ileocolonoscopy are part of the investigation of new IBD and are also used for disease surveillance, particularly in those who are not responding well to their medical treatment.
- To investigate symptoms of gastro-oesophageal reflux disease (GORD) resistant to treatment: oesophageal pH monitoring gives a picture of the severity of acid reflux, but OGD is recommended for those resistant to or dependent on proton pump inhibitors for histological examination and to look for other possible diagnoses.
- As part of the assessment and treatment of chronic liver disease and oesophageal varices: variceal bleeding is the commonest cause of severe haematemesis in children; OGD is used to grade the severity of the varices, to band varices where there has been bleeding and sometimes to repeat banding.

Table I Indications for oesophagogastroduodenoscopy (OGD)

Diagnostic OGD needed	Diagnostic OGD may be needed	Therapeutic OGD needed
Confirmation of coeliac disease	Vomiting	Gastrointestinal bleeding
Possible inflammatory bowel disease	Weight loss	Caustic or foreign body ingestion
Assessment of liver disease	Anaemia	Banding of varices
Gastro-oesophageal reflux disease	Malabsorptive chronic diarrhoea	Dilatation of stricture
	Dysphagia	
	Recurrent abdominal pain	

▷ Contraindications

There are few absolute contraindications to OGD in those whom the anaesthetist considers fit for an anaesthetic. These include: intestinal perforation and cervical trauma, and absence of informed consent or the relevant competent professional.

▷ Equipment

There is a choice of endoscopes to suit the size of patient. All have an instrument channel, and accessory channels to insufflate air or inject or aspirate water. The appropriate environment and standard approach are illustrated in the CD.

Pitfalls

- Anaesthetic risk applies to all anaesthetic procedures.
- Perforation and bleeding are rare, but may follow biopsy in the severely malnourished infant.
- Inadequately trained endoscopists should always be expertly supervised.
- Poor-quality biopsies of insufficient number (e.g. in possible coeliac disease due to patchy nature of the changes), may lead to a false negative result.

▷ Results and their interpretation

Results from an OGD consist of:

- Macroscopic findings – a description is written, photos can be taken and the video can also be recorded and kept for future reference.
- Histology – gives most information.
- Other results such as those of *Helicobacter pylori* testing or disaccharidase levels in biopsy material.

Some of the commonest diagnoses are listed below together with the macroscopic and microscopic findings:

- **Coeliac disease**: sometimes villous atrophy is noticeable with the naked eye, but the diagnosis is made on histological findings of duodenal villous blunting or atrophy, and increased intraepithelial lymphocytes. The changes can be patchy and therefore four duodenal biopsies are needed.
- **IBD**: Crohn's disease produces changes that are patchy not just macroscopically but microscopically, with non-caseating granulomas in a small percentage, and significant inflammation in the stomach, oesophagus or duodenum. Macroscopic changes can range from mild erythema or nodularity of the stomach to more obvious features such as ulceration or cobblestoning. Some children with Crohn's disease have changes on OGD changes but normal findings on colonoscopy. Ulcerative colitis was originally thought not to affect the gastrointestinal tract outside the colon, but more recently changes have been documented in OGD such as mild non-specific gastritis.
- **GORD**: this has macroscopic changes ranging from normal or mild erythema to more obvious erosions affecting much of the oesophageal circumference. In children more severe changes are rare. In all cases biopsy is mandatory, which may show basal zone hyperplasia, or inflammatory infiltrate of epithelium or lamina propria consisting of polymorphs and some eosinophils. (The presence of very large numbers of eosinophils per high power field raises the possibility of eosinophilic oesophagitis.) *Helicobacter* may be detected by using a campylobacter-like organism (CLO) test on one of the biopsies, and it can also be seen on histology (especially with methylene blue stain). The CLO test uses the fact that the *H. pylori* metabolises urea to ammonia (using its urease activity), the pH of the medium rises and the pH-sensitive phenol dye turns the medium bright pink/red.
- Other causes for epigastric pain may be found, such as erosions or even ulcers.

▷ **Further reading**

Gershman G, Ament M (eds). *Practical Pediatric Gastrointestinal Endoscopy*. Oxford: Wiley-Blackwell Publishing, 2007.

Walker AW, Kleinman RE, Sherman PM *et al.* (eds). *Pediatric Gastrointestinal Disease*, 4th edn. Philadelphia: BC Decker, 2004.

OESOPHAGOGASTRODUODENOSCOPY

▶ Background

Gastrostomy refers to an opening into the stomach created surgically for the purpose of nutritional support or decompression of the gastrointestinal tract.

▷ Indications

A gastrostomy becomes necessary when adequate nutrition cannot be provided orally despite the presence of a functioning gastrointestinal tract. In the short term, this problem can be overcome by placement of a nasogastric or nasojejunal tube. However, in the long term, such as in terms of months to years, most patients and parents prefer to have a gastrostomy.

- The most common reason for creation of a gastrostomy is neurological or muscular impairment where swallowing is affected to such a degree that oral feeding is unsafe (due to risk of aspiration) or is ineffective (adequate nutrition cannot be maintained).
- Children with chronic illness such as malignancy, renal failure (poor appetite) or cystic fibrosis (increased requirement) may need nutritional supplements. This may be administered as overnight feeds through a gastrostomy leaving the daytime free for normal activity.
- Oral feeding may not be possible due to anatomical factors such as in oesophageal atresia or oesophageal stricture.
- In severe oesophageal injury the oesophagus may have to be 'rested' to allow it to heal and prevent mediastinitis. Such injury could be the result of corrosive ingestion, foreign body or medical intervention.

▷ Types of gastrostomy

Classically, gastrostomies have been classified as permanent or temporary. A permanent gastrostomy involves creation of a tube with the stomach wall (Janeway) and joining stomach mucosa to skin similar to a bowel stoma. As this type of gastrostomy is lined by mucosa, it will not close spontaneously – hence the term permanent. However, creation of this type of gastrostomy is very rare.

Practically all gastrostomies are temporary, i.e. the track between the skin and the stomach is lined by granulation tissue and is held open by a tube. Removal of the tube usually results in rapid and spontaneous closure of the gastrostomy track. Such a gastrostomy may be created by open surgery, endoscopically or under radiological guidance.

Open gastrostomy

This procedure involves laparotomy via a vertical or transverse upper abdominal incision. An appropriate site for the gastrostomy is identified depending on anatomy and likely further reconstruction. The gastrostomy tube is inserted through the centre of two concentric purse-string sutures (Stamm). The tube exits via the abdominal wall and the stomach is hitched to the parietal peritoneum. This procedure may be the only option in conditions such as oesophageal atresia, oesophageal stricture or injury.

Percutaneous endoscopic gastrostomy

Percutaneous endoscopic gastrostomy (PEG) is commonly performed by the 'pull' technique. In this procedure, an endoscope is inserted into the stomach, internal anatomy is identified and the stomach is inflated. A cannula is introduced at an appropriate location through the abdominal wall into the stomach. A wire is passed into the stomach via the cannula, which is grasped endoscopically and delivered through the mouth. The gastrostomy tube is attached to the wire and pulled through into the stomach. A flange at the end of the tube prevents extrusion and holds the stomach against the abdominal wall until the track 'matures'.

Percutaneous endoscopic gastrostomy may not be possible in case of unfavourable anatomy such as when the stomach is high up under the rib cage or there is a large overlying liver. A serious complication of the procedure is inadvertent passage of the cannula through another viscus. Typically the transverse colon is involved and as transfixation is eccentric, the problem may not be identified until much later when a gastrocolic fistula develops. One should therefore have a high index of suspicion with regard to gastrocolic fistula if a patient who has had a PEG suddenly develops profuse watery diarrhoea that resembles feeds. A gastrogram will demonstrate the problem.

Laparoscopy-assisted percutaneous endoscopic gastrostomy

A laparoscopic port is created at the umbilicus and PEG is carried out under direct vision. The risk of damage to other viscera is therefore minimised. If there is unfavourable anatomy, an additional port can be created to grasp the stomach and pull it to a more favourable location. This procedure is rapidly gaining popularity.

Gastrostomy feeds are commonly commenced 24 hours after placement of a new PEG after an initial trial of clear fluid. However, there is evidence to suggest that feeds may be safely commenced as early as 4 hours after the procedure. There are smaller reports of immediate postoperative feeding as well.

▷ Gastrostomy care

The site should be kept clean with sterile water and gauze. Creams, powders and occlusive dressings should be avoided. Immersive baths should be encouraged to allow crusts to loosen and a track to form.

The gastrostomy must be rotated by one complete circle daily to ensure mobility and detect migration. From 10 days after the procedure, the fixator may be loosened to allow cleaning under. The tube should be moved in a short distance (about 1 cm) and pulled back out and rotated at the same time.

The skin around the stoma should be inspected daily for discharge, redness, bleeding, leakage and breakdown. There is no requirement to restrict activity. Children with a gastrostomy are allowed to lie on their front or crawl. They can go swimming, although the site must be thoroughly cleaned and dried afterwards.

Feeds

Feeds should be carried out in the upright, sitting position or in mother's arms. The position is maintained for at least 45 minutes after the feed. Feeding is made as much like a family meal as possible. Infants are given a pacifier at the same time to promote sucking and to associate this with gastric filling.

Helpful hints

Common problems and how to deal with:
- Discharge: some clear or seropurulent discharge is commonly seen around gastrostomy sites. This is due to local reaction to the tube. Dried exudate forms crusts which should be cleaned away regularly. Staining of clothes by the discharge may be troublesome.

- Infection: purulent discharge associated with pain, tenderness and surrounding erythema suggests infection. A swab is taken and initial treatment with flucloxacillin is commenced.
- Overgranulation: troublesome overgranulation causes bleeding and discharge. This may be dealt with by chemocautery of the excessive granulation tissue using silver nitrate sticks. The procedure is painless as granulation tissue does not have nerve endings.
- Blockage of tube: this is avoided by flushing the tube with a small amount of water after every feed. Blocked tubes may be cleared by a commercially available preparation of pancreatic enzymes. Alternatives are pineapple juice and cola.
- Accidental dislodgement: if the tube is pulled out accidentally, the track may close within a few hours. An alternative tube such as a nasogastric tube must be inserted via the opening and taped until the gastrostomy can be replaced.
- Leakage of gastric content: gastric content is highly irritant and leakage around the tube leads to rapid skin breakdown. Leakage may be due to a loose fixation or an inadequately inflated balloon. Placement of the tube in a skinfold may also be associated with leakage. This can be prevented by preoperative marking and avoiding overfeeding. If the track has enlarged due to excessive movement of the device or infection, a period with a smaller-bore tube *in situ* will allow the track to reduce in diameter.

▷ **Button gastrostomy**

A button gastrostomy is a simple skin level device with a one way valve and a retaining device – usually a balloon. A detachable connecting tube is used to feed and is removed at the end and stored until next use. A PEG can be changed for a button device once the track has adequately matured, i.e. no sooner than 3 weeks.

▶ Indication

To obtain a sterile urine specimen for culture in infants and children less than 2 years old. (If the child is older than 2 years, sterile urine should be collected by urethral catheterisation.)

▷ Procedure

Position the child in a supine position and hold their legs apart. Restrain the child firmly. Select a puncture site in the midline of the abdomen, approximately 1–2 cm above the superior edge of the pubic bone.

Prepare the skin by cleaning it with chlorhexidine antiseptic solution and then place a 22 gauge needle at the planned puncture site, perpendicular to the plane of the abdominal wall, which is usually 10–20 degrees from the true vertical position.

Pierce the skin and advance the syringe gently aspirating at the same time. If urine is not obtained, instead of removing the needle and starting again, repeat the technique but at a different angle.

▷ Complications

- Haematuria: microscopic haematuria is very common but self-limiting and of no consequence
- Intestinal perforation: this is fortunately very rare
- Infection: infection of the abdominal wall is possible if the sterile technique was not adequate

Helpful hints

- Ask an assistant to occlude the penile urethra in a male infant to prevent urination, while preparations are being made.
- It is also wise to wait for at least an hour after the last void before attempting the procedure.

▶ Background

Bladder cathererisation is commonly used in critically ill children in order to measure urine output in the management of fluid balance

▷ Indications

- Any child requiring intensive care
- Multiple trauma particularly involving the abdomen
- Postoperative management of a patient in whom the catheter helps in the management of the child's fluid balance
- Acute urinary retention
- Severe head trauma
- Shock
- To obtain a urinary specimen
- Intermittent catheterisation in children with underlying neurological problems such as spina bifida

▷ Procedure

The patient must remain still during the procedure, by gentle restraint if necessary.

1. Wear sterile gloves.
2. Prepare the urethral meatus and the penis or the perineal area with chlorhexidine antiseptic solution.
3. A Foley catheter of the most appropriate seize must be selected (8 Fr for newborns, 10 Fr for most children and 12 Fr for older children).
4. Inflate the balloon on the catheter with sterile water or normal saline to test its competence.
5. Lubricate the catheter tip with sterile lubricant to prevent trauma.

For the male child:

1. Gently grasp and extend the penile shaft to straighten out the urethra.
2. Hold the catheter near the distal tip and advance it up the urethra, unless resistance or an obstruction is encountered. If this occurs repeat the procedure with a smaller catheter. Feeding tubes can also be used as urinary catheters but do not seem to function as well.
3. When the catheter reaches the junction of the penile shaft and perineum it may help to position the penis more vertically.
4. The catheter should be passed all the way until the Y junction of the catheter since urine will flow even while the catheter is in the urethra and if the balloon is inflated in the urethra it might lead to trauma and bleeding. The catheter should be taped to the child's leg, leaving a lax portion to cater for movement of the child. The balloon must be inflated when the catheter is in place and deflated before removal.

For the female child: the principles are similar.

1. Spread the labia fully in order to visualise the urethra.
2. Insert the well lubricated pre-tested Foley catheter up to the Y junction, well into the bladder.
3. Inflate the balloon and secure along the side of the leg as previously described.

▷ Contraindications

- An anatomical abnormality such as hypospadias or epispadias might make catheterisation difficult.
- A gross coagulopathy should be corrected before catheter insertion just in case it is difficult.

Helpful hints

- Do not force the catheter.
- Always reassess the need for the catheter to be left *in situ* because of associated urinary infections, e.g. with Gram-negative organisms and *Candida*.

► Background

Acute renal failure (ARF) is the sudden loss of the ability of the kidneys to excrete waste, concentrate urine and conserve electrolytes. In terms of urine output, the definition used in children is a sustained reduction in urine output from 1 mL/kg/h to less than 0.5 mL/kg/h.

Acute renal failure is seen in approximately 10 per cent of critically ill children and when combined with respiratory failure has mortality greater than 50 per cent.

▷ Pathophysiology

Acute renal failure can be divided into three types:

- pre-renal
- intra-renal (intrinsic)
- post-renal (obstructive)

Pre-renal is caused by a decrease of renal perfusion and is the most common type of ARF. The decrease in renal perfusion is usually secondary to a reduction in cardiac output, i.e. shocked states, but it can also be due to occlusion of the renal artery through spasm or extrinsic compression. Renal function is impaired but renal parenchyma is preserved, and thus function can be restored by restoring renal perfusion. Intra-renal failure is due to acute tubular necrosis (ATN), nephrotoxic drugs or severe unrelieved pre-renal oliguria. Post-renal failure is caused by obstruction of the flow of urine leading to back pressure and parenchymal damage.

▷ Investigations to differentiate the cause of acute renal failure

- Urinalysis (Table 1).
- Fractional excretion of sodium <1 per cent = pre-renal failure and >2.5 per cent = intrinsic renal failure. Not always especially on diuretic therapy.
- Imaging – ultrasound is preferred as it avoids contrast media.
- Renal biopsy – indicated in unknown cause or delayed recovery.

Table 1 Urinalysis in acute renal failure

Urinalysis	Pre-renal	Renal
Specific gravity	High >1.020	Fixed 1.010
Sodium	Low <20	High >40
Urine/plasma (U/P) urea	High 20	Low 10
U/P creatinine	High 40	Low 10
U/P osmolality	High 2.1	Low 1.2
Osmolality	High	Low
Sediment	Normal	Cells and casts: • Granular and epithelial – acute tubular necrosis • White cell or eosinophilic – acute interstitial nephritis • Red cell and proteinuria – acute glomerulonephritis or vasculitis

▷ **Management of acute renal failure**

Maximising the delivery of oxygen to the tissues by optimising the respiratory function and cardiac output is the first step in trying to protect/restore renal function. Often during the recovery stage there is polyuria. It is important to keep up with the diuresis and ensure adequate circulating volume.

Avoid fluid overload after initial resuscitation by fluid restriction, i.e. aiming to balance insensible losses of 400 mL/m^2/day plus ongoing losses. Avoid drugs that are metabolised by the kidneys, but if unavoidable their doses and frequencies should be altered.

▷ **Indications**

- Renal failure with any of the following:
  - uncontrolled hyperkalaemia
  - uncontrolled symptomatic acidosis
  - fluid overload
  - uraemic symptoms, i.e. encephalopathy
- Tumour lysis syndrome

Box 1 Complications of renal replacement therapy

Haemodialysis
- Hypotension
- Bleeding
- Hypoxaemia
- Cramps
- Leukopenia
- Arrhythmias
- Infection
- Pyrogen reactions
- Dialysis disequilibrium syndrome
- Access problems (blood)
- Technical mishaps

Haemofiltration
- Bleeding
- Thrombosis of haemofilter
- Technical mishaps
- Haemolysis
- Access problems (blood)
- Hypotension
- Line infection

Peritoneal dialysis
- Peritonitis
- Catheter infections
- Catheter dysfunction
- Abdominal pain
- Respiratory failure with splinting of the diaphragm
- Visceral perforation
- Pleural effusion
- Technical mishaps

ACUTE RENAL FAILURE (HAEMODIALYSIS/FILTRATION AND PERITONEAL DIALYSIS)

- Manipulation of metabolic environment
- Drug intoxication
- Rhabdomyolysis
- Possible removal of toxins or inflammatory cytokines

There is some suggestion that filtration in particular may remove inflammatory mediators that contribute to cardiovascular compromise in sepsis.

In the intensive care unit, the majority of patients are haemodynamically unstable and haemofiltration or peritoneal dialysis (PD) have been the therapies of choice in this setting. The major advantage of PD is that it does not require vascular access which is often the limiting factor in haemofiltration. Also, PD can be performed with less experience and monitoring, making it more suitable for a wider range of hospital environments. The decision on which mode to use is often based on the previous experience of the unit, however, known complications (Box 1) should be taken into consideration.

▷ Haemofiltration and haemodiafiltration

Haemofiltration is the removal of plasma water by the filtration of blood. The biochemistry is controlled by removing large volumes of filtrate and replacing it with electrolyte containing fluid. The more filtrate removed and replaced the more efficient the process. The transport of the molecules is achieved by convection (Figure 1). In addition for any given filtration rate a higher clearance of solute can be obtained by pre-dilution, although post-dilution uses less replacement fluid. Pre-dilution also extends circuit life. Remember that solutes are distributed in both the intracellular and extracellular compartments thus the volume of filtration necessary to control biochemistry relates to total body water. Clinical experience has shown that a replacement of approximately 50 per cent of body weight is usually adequate for solute and electrolyte removal. With total pre-dilution approx 25 per cent of replacement fluid is lost in ultrafiltrate so an equivalent increase in replacement fluid is needed. The

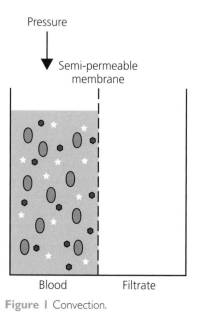

Figure 1 Convection.

newer machinery has the ability to mix pre- and post-dilution, which may negate the need to increase the rate.

Continuous dialysis works by running a counter current flow of dialysis fluid to blood flow resulting in a gradient. Molecules flow down the gradient resulting in excess electrolytes entering the dialysis fluid or in to the blood (diffusion). Relatively low dialysate flow rates can be generated by continuous therapy limiting the clearance, however dialysis is a more efficient method of removing urea, creatinine and drugs.

Both methods can be run together or separately using the same filter. The major limiting step for either is the availability of good central venous access to allow the high blood flow necessary to prevent clotting of the filter and usefully filtration/dialysis. Remember a low blood flow rate, high haematocrit and high plasma concentration will limit the rate at which filtration can occur and solutes are removed.

Procedure

The first step is the insertion of a vascular catheter. This is normally a double lumen line. Table 2 gives some suggestions for size selection. Although the radius is the main factor in resistance, length does have an impact. Even with a large cannula, there can be flow problems and these can often be improved by rotation or slight retraction of the cannula.

Table 2 Cannula size

Weight (kg)	Size (fg)
3–10	6.5
10–20	8
20–50	11
>50	12

▷ Replacement fluids

A large range of replacement fluids are available, with buffering based on lactate or bicarbonate. In the paediatric intensive care unit (PICU), bicarbonate has become the first choice as lactate is often one of the waste products renal replacement therapy is commenced to remove. Furthermore, the replacement fluids can have varying concentrations of electrolytes. If a rapid drop in potassium is required, bags with no potassium are available, but in general it is safer to use fluid with 4 mmol/L potassium. If the patient is very hypernatraemic, i.e. Na >160 mmol/L, sodium can be added to the bags to reduce the speed of sodium reduction.

Once the circuit is primed and the access obtained, the starting parameters have to be considered (Table 3). However, every child is different and thus individual tailoring

Table 3 Initial parameters

Filtration	30 mL/kg/h	This will exchange about 50% body weight in 24 h
Dialysate flow rate	20 mL/kg/h	Maximal efficacy is achieved at two to three times the blood flow rate
Fluid loss	Individualise	This is the net fluid loss through haemofiltration and will depend on the child's needs. It is practically difficult to achieve a negative balance of more than 5–10% of the patient's body weight in 24 h
Blood flow	6–9 mL/kg/min	This is at least 10 × filtration rate and prevents excessive haemoconcentration in the filter

will be required. In particular some patients require high-volume treatment, i.e. patients with metabolic diseases, sepsis and drug removal. Remember that in high-volume treatment, dramatic effects on electrolyte balance can occur, thus frequent review of potassium, phosphate, calcium, sodium and pH is essential.

As mentioned one of the problems with haemofiltration is the potential for clotting of the circuit. In the UK, anticoagulation is most commonly achieved using unfractionated heparin. Heparin is also used during priming to coat the lines and filter. Prior to connection the patient is given a loading dose of up to 50 U/kg followed by a continuous infusion of 0–30 U/kg/h with an aim to achieve an activated clotting time (ACT) between 120 and 180 seconds, or an activated partial prothrombin time of 1.2 to 1.5 times the respective baseline value. Other agents may be used, such as prostaglandin and sodium citrate.

When the renal replacement first starts there is often an initial hypotensive period. The reasons are multifactorial: the circuit itself produces an inflammatory response; there is an additional circulating volume placing more strain on the heart; transient reduction of serum inotropic levels. In very small patients the circuit will often need to be blood primed to prevent haemodilution.

▷ Peritoneal dialysis

Peritoneal dialysis is still widely used as a renal replacement therapy for children. It also has a role in paediatric intensive care, in particular in the postoperative cardiac patient, where the placement of a PD catheter can be done under direct visualisation in theatre. The main advantage is that no intravenous access is required and it can be used in infants with weights <2 kg. It remains the cheapest and simplest to perform and is usable in low cardiac output states. It is effective in many situations, however, there are recognised contraindications:

- Diaphragmatic hernia
- Omphalocoele
- Gastroschisis
- Possibility of intra-abdominal catastrophe
- Recent abdominal surgery
- Multiple adhesions
- Peritonitis
- Presence of ventriculoperitoneal shunt

In PD, the peritoneum acts as a semi-permeable membrane. Solute exchange takes place by means of three forces: diffusion, convection and osmosis. The main osmotic agent in PD is glucose, thus as the glucose concentration of the fluid is increased, so does the efficacy of fluid removal (Figure 2). The other parameters that need to be set after choosing the dialysis fluid are the fluid volume instilled into the peritoneum per cycle, time allowed for the fluid to drain into the abdomen, dwell time when the PD fluid is left *in situ* and drain time. The fluid volume and dwell time affect fluid removal (Figure 3) and solute removal (Figure 4).

As glucose is the main osmotic agent, increasing the glucose concentration from 1.5 per cent to 4.5 per cent will increase the amount of fluid that drains out, thereby playing a crucial role in managing the fluid balance. The glucose concentration should be the minimum possible to allow the correct fluid removal. The higher the concentration the more likely the patient is to become hyperglycaemic. Higher glucose concentrations are also thought to irritate the peritoneum.

The starting fill volume should be 10–15 mL/kg and this can be slowly increased to

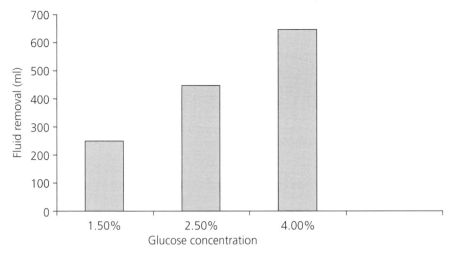

Figure 2 Fluid removal related to glucose concentration in PD fluid.

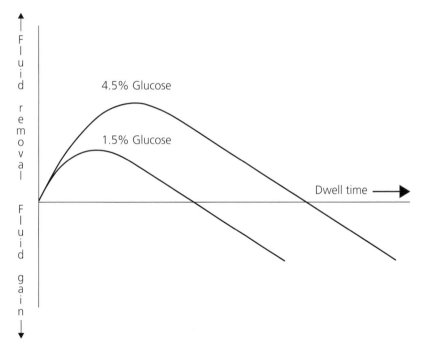

Figure 3 Fluid removal: relationship to dwell time and glucose concentration.

a maximum of 50 mL/kg to increase diffusion and thus improve the efficiency of the dialysis. Remember the larger the fill volume the more likely there will be respiratory and cardiovascular instability. The filling usually occurs over a 10-minute period and then an initial dwell time of 30–60 minutes. The fluid is then drained over a 10-minute period, although if fluid is still draining at the end of 10 minutes continue until draining stops. If more fluid removal is required dwell time can be reduced to 10–30 minutes with increased frequency of cycles. In neonates the response to dwell time is very variable and therefore alternative strategies may have to be used.

ACUTE RENAL FAILURE (HAEMODIALYSIS/FILTRATION AND PERITONEAL DIALYSIS)

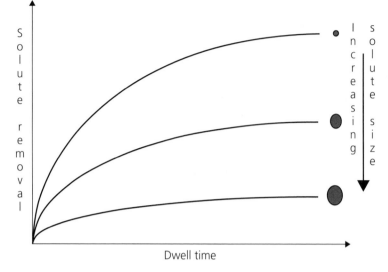

Figure 4 Solute clearance.

In situations where a 'full' abdomen cannot be tolerated it is possible to insert two PD catheters, thus allowing cross-flow. In cross-flow, the same fill volumes are used, but the fluid is infused over 1 hour rather than 10 minutes while at the same time it is drained from the other catheter.

▷ Buffers

Bicarbonate is often part of the dialysate fluid and acts as a buffer, given that these patients often have multiorgan failure and are acidotic. Previously, lactate-based fluids were used for buffering, however more recently, bicarbonate is increasingly used (Table 4).

Table 4 Advantages and disadvantages of bicarbonated fluid

Advantages of bicarbonate	Disadvantages of bicarbonate
Does not need to be metabolised	Less stable than lactate-based fluids
Can be used in liver failure	Must be mixed before use
Can be used with high serum lactate	
Theoretically quicker improvement in acidosis	
Licensed for use in children	
Reduced inflow pain	

PD fluid bags often have additives, the most common being heparin and antibiotics. Heparin is used to try to prevent fibrin deposits from blocking the PD catheters and up to 500 IU/L has been used. This should be used with caution in small infants, as absorption of the heparin may occur in sufficient quantities to cause deranged clotting.

Helpful hints

- Leakage around the catheter site is a common problem, although less so in tunnelled catheters. If there is a leak it needs to be reduced to a minimum as it increases the risk of infection as well leading to difficulties in working out input/output and fluid balance. One method is to try re-suturing around the insertion site, or alternatively using fibrin glue.
- Poor drainage is the most frequent cause of failure of PD. Flushing the catheter and preventing fibrin accumulation by increasing the heparin dosage and/or urokinase can be attempted. A plain abdominal X-ray is rarely justified as it is unlikely to demonstrate the cause and in many cases catheter relocation will be required.
- Peritonitis is a major concern in PD as it can be life-threatening. The standard symptoms of pain, fever and cloudy PD fluid do not have to be present; in fact up to 6 per cent of culture-positive adults do not have cloudy PD fluid. Local guidelines should be developed with the microbiology department before starting.
- Finally, complications encountered following the insertion of the PD catheter need to be considered. Insertion by direct vision during cardiac operations or by a general surgeon provides less risk of perforation, however, bedside insertion in experienced hands has been shown to be safe and avoids a general anaesthetic. The PD catheters are best tunnelled with two cuffs to reduce the problem of site leakage and if possible left *in situ* for 2 weeks prior to use, although in the intensive care unit this is rarely possible. Direct percutaneous insertion with Seldinger's technique can be used in acute situations, but it is associated with a higher risk of complications. If this technique is used the bladder should be empty and the patient should not be constipated. If there is already fluid in the abdomen then ultrasound guidance should be used. The skin in the chosen site should be pinched to allow the needle to be inserted and then removed quickly to avoid perforation.

In summary, PD remains a useful therapy in acute renal failure, although its use is decreasing.

URINE EXAMINATION: BAG SPECIMEN

▶ Background

Urine examination is an important part of the screening of any infant or child with pyrexia, unexplained vomiting or failure to thrive. The symptoms of urine infections can vary from overt symptoms of dysuria in the older child to non-specific symptoms of poor feeding, lethargy and irritability in the newborn and infant.

Due to the high frequency and potentially serious nature of urinary tract infections particularly in newborns and infants, urine screening for urinary tract infection is a very important and early part of the work up of a child who is unwell and has presented without obvious localising signs.

▷ Indications

- The diagnosis of urinary tract infections which depends on the culture of bacteria from the urine

In addition, urine can be collected for the following purposes:

- To check for the presence of sugar, acetone, blood, ketones cells, casts bacteria or crystals and to facilitate a urine dipstick looking for evidence of infection
- To aid in the diagnosis of renal abnormalities
- To determine effectiveness of therapy by measuring pH and specific gravity

An accurate diagnosis may be difficult to establish owing to frequent contamination of voided specimens, hence when planning a urine examination in order to avoid contamination, the following should be available:

- Sterile water
- Antiseptic solution such as povidone iodine, chlorhexidine or soap
- Sterile cotton balls
- Urine collector
- Specimen container
- Non-sterile gloves

▷ Methods of collection

There are four common methods of collection of urine for testing. However before collection, it is worth remembering that the groin is a warm moist area that harbours numerous bacteria which are normal skin commensals.

In order to avoid bacterial contamination, which would render the urine examination unreliable, it is important to disinfect the area surrounding the uretheral meatus. This can be done as described above with povidone iodine, chlorhexidine or indeed soap and water.

Urine bag collection

In neonates and infants and those toddlers who have not been potty trained, the application of an adhesive sterile bag on the groin area around the respective meatus can be a useful method of diagnosing urinary tract infections.

■ Method

After explaining the urine collection procedure to the child and family, place the child in a frog leg position so that the genitalia are exposed

Wash your hands, put gloves on and cleanse the genitalia as follows:

Male

Wipe the tip of the penis with a cotton ball and soap solution or gauze in a circular motion downwards and outwards towards the scrotum. Repeat the procedure with sterile water and allow to air dry before applying the sterile bag.

Female

Wipe the labia majora with cleansing solution from top to bottom, i.e. clitoris to anus. Then spread the labia majora apart, wiping the labia minora in the same manner and then wipe down with a cotton ball dipped in sterile water.

In the male, the penis is placed in the plastic bag and the adhesive surface is applied to the surrounding skin; in the female the opening of the bag is placed around the external genitalia.

Care must be taken to transfer the urine specimen to a sterile pot without any contamination.

The other methods of urine sample collection are direct urinary catherisation and, in infants, suprapubic aspiration. In toilet trained children, a midstream urine culture obtained after cleaning the urethral meatus and retracting the foreskin in a male or parting the labia in the female should provide adequate asepsis and avoid contamination.

URINE EXAMINATION: BAG SPECIMEN

▶ # Background

In order to maintain tight glucose control and to titrate the dose of insulin, diabetic patients must undertake regular monitoring of blood glucose levels. Blood glucose monitoring identifies variations in blood control and allows the patient to adjust insulin requirements on a day-to-day basis. Ideally testing should be done four times a day. If using an insulin pump, six times a day is a minimum. The aim is to record a blood glucose level throughout a whole day. In order to obtain a sample of blood the patient has to use a lancet device to pierce the skin and squeeze out a drop of blood for the blood glucose meter to analyse.

▷ # Indications/contraindications

Every patient with diabetes needs to check their blood sugar regularly. There are no exceptions. A relative contraindication is extreme needle phobia and this should be recognised as a barrier to testing. This can be overcome on an intermittent basis with the use of a continuous blood glucose monitor (CGMS), which constantly records the blood sugar via a subcutaneous cannula. The use of CGMS as a first-line method of recording blood glucose is not standard practice. Devices such as indirect measurement (e.g. infrared devices) are not yet accurate enough for use in practice.

▷ # Blood glucose meters

Blood glucose testing utilises the glucose oxidase reaction, and some use glucose dehydrogenase. The oxidation process product generates a potential difference across the test strip, which is measured and reported as a numerical value. The vast majority of testing is blood spot analysis. Glucose can be measured in other fluids, but these are not used in day-to-day management of diabetes. A recent advance has been the use of CGMS, which relies on a subcutaneous cannula measuring glucose level. This provides a reading continuously. Such a device can typically provide readings over a 3–4-day period before the cannula needs to be replaced.

There are many blood glucose monitors and finger prickers catering for all requirements (Tables 1 and 2). The meters need to be matched to the individual's needs. They differ in physical characteristics, volume of blood required, automated testing strips and speed of result. In addition, some meters now incorporate computer software packages to allow the patient and clinician to monitor and analyse blood control in more detail with data transmission to computers. Table 1 lists the meters currently available in the UK. Availability may vary depending on country of origin and new products on the market.

Preparation

Before obtaining a sample the patient should wash and dry their hands. An alcohol wipe can alter the reading so, if used, the finger should be thoroughly dried. The patient then uses a lancet inserted into a finger pricker to obtain a blood sample (Figure 1). Ideally, the sample should be taken from the side of the finger pulp and a different finger used each time, as this will hurt less. If the blood does not come, the patient should warm their hands, or hold their arm downward to allow flow of blood to the periphery. The finger is gently squeezed, and the test strip applied to the blood drop. The blood is drawn onto the testing strip by capillary action. As detailed above the result is calculated within a few seconds. Some meters allow alternative site testing but be aware that glucose ranges can vary across the body, particularly if the drop in glucose level is large. There are no standards of normal glucose ranges for alternative sites.

Table 1 Glucose meters

Manufacturer	Meter	Volume of blood required (µL)	Time for tests (/sec)	Data downloading
Abbott Diabetes Care	Optium Xceed	0.6	5	Yes
	Medisense Optium	5.0	30	Yes
	Medisense soft-sense	3.0	20	
	Freestyle	0.3	15	
	Freestyle Mini	0.3	7	
	Freestyle Freedom	0.3	5	
Bayer Healthcare	Ascensia Contour	0.6	15	
	Ascensia Breeze	2.0–3.0	30	
BBI Healthcare	SensoCard test strip	0.5	5	
Home Diagnostics	Prestige QX smart system	4.0	Up to 50	
	True track smart system	1.0	10	
Hypo Guard	Supreme Plus	4.0	30–60	
LifeScan	Onetouch ultra	1.0	5	
	Onetouch ultra 2	1.0	5	
	Onetouch ultra smart	1.0	5	
	Onetouch ultraeasy	1.0	5	
Menarini Diagnostics	Glucomen Visio	0.8	10	
	Glucomen PC	2.0	30	
Roche Diagnostics	Accu-chek Compact Plus	1.5	5	Yes
	Accu-chek Aviva	0.6	5	

Table 2 Finger prickers

Manufacturer	Device	Lancets
Abbott Diabetes Care	Easytouch Freestyle	Ascensia Microlet, BD Microfine+ 30G, BD Microfine 33G, Cleanlet fine, finepoint,
Bayer Healthcare	Ascensia Microlet Ascensia Vaculance	freestyle, Glucomen fine, Hypo Guard supreme, Palco autolancet, Medisense Fine,
BD Medical–Diabetes	BD Optimus Hypolance	Milward Sterilet, Monolet, Monolet Extra, Onetouch Ultrasoft, Unilet Comfortouch,
Hypo Guard	Onetouch Ultrasoft	Unilet General Purpose, Unilet General
LifeScan	Glucolet Dual	Purpose Superlite, Vitrex Soft, Glucomen
Menarini	Monojector	Visio Sensors
Tyco		
Roche Diagnostics	Accu-chek Softclix Accu-chek Multiclix	Softclix lancets, Multiclix lancet (six lancets in a drum)
Home Diagnostics	Prestige Smart system Gentle Draw	Ascensia Microlet, BD Microfine+ 30G, BD Microfine 33G, Cleanlet fine, finepoint, freestyle, Glucomen fine, Hypo Guard supreme, Medisense Thin, Milward Sterilet, Monolet, Monolet Extra, Onetouch Ultrasoft, Unilet Comfortouch, Unilet General Purpose, Unilet General Purpose Superlite, Vitrex Soft

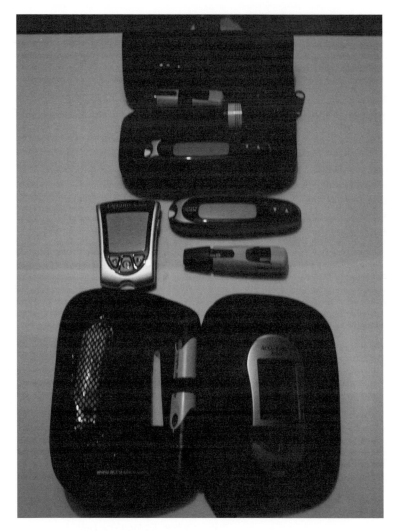

Figure 1 Equipment for blood glucose monitoring.

Pitfalls

- Overestimation of blood glucose as a result of: glucose contamination of fingers; or dirt on the monitor screens obscuring the reading (it does happen).
- Underestimation of blood glucose as a result of: inadequate blood sample; blood applied too late; contamination of the testing site (water or saliva on the finger); or excessive squeezing of the fingers.
- Extremes of temperatures leading to glucose monitor malfunction.
- The wrong units of blood glucose on the meter (set as mg/dL instead of mmol/L).
- The incorrect date and time set on the meter leading to an incorrect record of the blood glucose.
- Deliberate false record of blood glucose (diary different from machine readings).
- Infrequent blood glucose testing leading to an insufficient record of the blood glucose trends.

▷ Results and interpretation

Blood glucose levels are calibrated to a standard for each meter. The mechanism for this varies. Some require a numeric code to be entered against each new batch of testing strips, some calibrate against a standardised testing solution, and some are self-calibrating. The variability of readings is 10–15 per cent. Comparing different meters often results in different readings so is not advised for any one individual. Blood glucose levels are measured in mmol/L or as mg/dL. Day to day a patient aims for a serum blood glucose between 4 mmol/L and 7 mmol/L. A blood glucose >15 mmol/L will exceed the renal threshold and result in glycosuria. Persistent hyperglycaemia will eventually lead to ketoacidosis. Glucose <3.5 mmol/L leads to neuroglycopenia, an altered sensorium and a risk of seizure.

Patients are taught to adjust the dose of insulin in order to maintain their blood glucose levels between 4 mmol/L and 7 mmol/L. For glucose excursions, fast-acting insulin can be used to normalise a high glucose level, and carbohydrate can be ingested to correct a low level.

▷ Further reading

Hanas R. *Type 1 Diabetes in Children, Adolescents and Young Adults*, 3rd edn. London: Class Publishing, 2006.

Diabetes UK. The balance guide to testing and treating diabetes 2007. In: *Balance*. London: Diabetes UK.

► Background

Insulin administration provides an effective but not physiological replacement of absolute or relative insulinopenia. Replacement therapy started in 1922 following the discovery of insulin, and involved administering regular insulin before each main meal and one injection at night. With the advent of intermediate- and long-acting insulin and more recently analogue insulin, delivery can now be achieved in differing patterns with the aim of mimicking physiological insulin secretion.

▷ Indications

The indications for administration of insulin are:

- In type 1 diabetes – absolute or relative insulinopenia required to maintain normal glucose homeostasis.
- In type 2 diabetes – where insulin-sensitising agents are insufficient to maintain normal glucose homeostasis.

▷ Contraindications

In confirmed type 1 diabetes almost every patient requires insulin. The exceptions are children in pre-diabetes before the onset of overt diabetes and children with very mild hyperglycaemia (particularly under 18 months of age) where the diagnosis of MODY (maturity onset diabetes of the young) should be considered. There are monogenic causes of diabetes, some of which can be treated with sulphonylureas, reducing or removing the need for insulin.

Generally patients with type 2 diabetes are non-insulin dependent at diagnosis but can acquire the need for insulin. In the advent of recurrent refractory hypoglycaemia the mode of delivery of insulin needs to be reconsidered. Finally, hyperglycaemia associated with infection, stress, drugs including steroid administration does not always require insulin therapy and is often transient.

▷ Equipment and materials

Administration of insulin requires the following:

- An insulin delivery device (Figure 1):
  - syringe
  - pen (pre-loaded with insulin – disposable; or insulin loaded as a cartridge – re-useable)
  - pump
  - inhaler (not licensed for paediatric use therefore not applicable here)
- Needles (dependent on type of delivery device)
- Recombinant human insulin (type and container)
- Consumables, if using an insulin pump (infusion set, needle introducer)

▷ Types of insulin (Figure 2)

- Rapid-acting: insulin lispro, insulin aspart and insulin glulisine
- Short-acting: regular (soluble) insulin
- Intermediate-acting: NPH (isophane) insulin
- Long-acting: insulin glargine and detemir

Combinations of the rapid- or short-acting insulin with the intermediate insulin are also available as premixed formulations. In addition it is possible to mix the rapid/short-acting and intermediate insulins within a syringe.

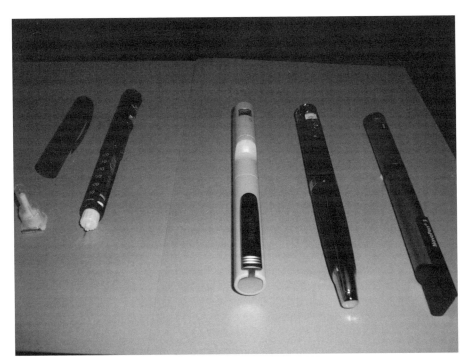

Figure 1 Types of insulin delivery system.

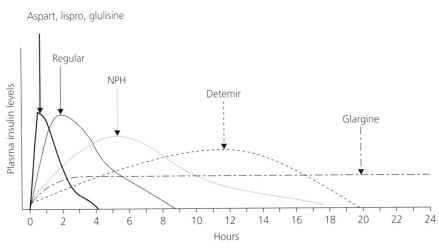

Figure 2 Time–action profiles of various types of insulin delivered as a subcutaneous injection.

▷ Regimens for delivery

- Once or twice daily injections of insulin delivered as intermediate- or long-acting or combinations of mixed insulin.
- Multiple daily injections (MDI) of insulin delivered as one long-acting injection and then injection of a fast-acting analogue insulin with each meal or significant snack.
- As a continuous subcutaneous infusion of insulin (CSII) delivered via an insulin pump.

There is no place for intermittent doses of short-acting insulin for long-term control of diabetes. Its use is in the management of acute hyperglycaemia as a rescue intervention to bring blood glucose into the normal range.

▷ Variations with age and situation

The insulin regimen has to be matched to the individual. The following factors need to be considered in deciding the appropriate device to use:

- age of the patient
- psychological factors
- lifestyle of the patient
- refractory hypoglycaemia
- intensity of treatment

At all ages of childhood there are different challenges when deciding on the right regimen.

- In early childhood a child eats frequently, erratically and has fluctuating levels of activity and therefore of glucose consumption. This leads to difficulties in accurately matching the dose of insulin to carbohydrate ingestion over a 24-hour period.
- Young adolescents strive for increased independence without necessarily the maturity to deliver insulin reliably out of parental control. They have increased variability of levels of exercise, sleep, energy use and compliance with medication. Once again this leads to greater variability in their glucose control.

The newer short-acting analogue insulins and CSII have allowed for much greater flexibility in delivery of insulin. The aim is to match insulin to the body's need. One must also always bear in mind the findings of the Diabetes Control and Complications Trial (DCCT) study (1995) which broadly showed that intensification of insulin treatment improved long-term glycaemic control, and reduced diabetes-related morbidity. This study has been the driving force in recent years towards intensification of regimens to deliver insulin (Figure 3).

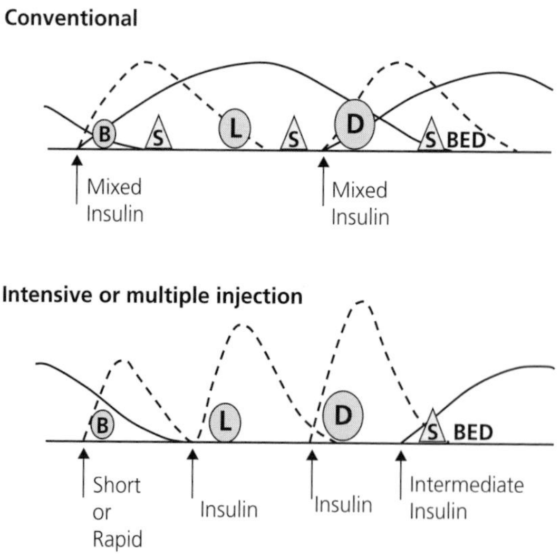

Conventional

Mixed Insulin — Mixed Insulin

Intensive or multiple injection

Short or Rapid — Insulin — Insulin — Intermediate Insulin

Figure 3 Relation of blood glucose, insulin and mealtimes (B, S, L and D corresponding to breakfast, snack, lunch and dinner). The dashed line represents insulin and the solid line represents blood glucose levels.

Pitfalls

The following are patterns not uncommonly seen in patients:

Hyperglycaemia
- Hyperglycaemia secondary to non-compliance with insulin therapy.
- The 'Dawn phenomenon', with high waking blood sugars as a result of relative insulin resistance in the early morning hours, caused by overnight growth hormone excretion.
- The Somogyi phenomenon, or rebound hyperglycaemia, with high waking blood sugars as a secondary consequence of overnight hypoglycaemia followed by a counter-regulatory hormonal response driving up blood sugars. This is more common in individuals on intermediate- or long-acting insulin (MDI and CSII regimens) and less common with twice-daily injections.
- Non-absorption of insulin due to: incorrect injection technique; injection into areas of lipohypertrophy; removal of the needle too early.
- Insulin delivery device failure (syringe, pen or pump).
- Non-compliance with medication.

Hypoglycaemia
- Nocturnal hypoglycaemia secondary to too much insulin before bedtime.
- Giving the wrong type insulin.
- After exercise, without reducing insulin or increasing carbohydrate intake.
- After alcohol use.

▷ Outcome

The gold standard for insulin treatment is the glycosylated haemoglobin (HbA1c) test. The test is based on the fact that glucose sticks to haemoglobin on red cells and the percentage of glycosylated haemoglobin reflects blood glucose levels over a 2–3-month period – the lifespan of a red cell (Table 1). As it is an average, it does not reflect the variability of glucose values. Remember that HbA1c is not reliable in a patient with a haemoglobinopathy (due to shorter lifespan of the red blood cell) in whom measurement of blood fructosamine level is an alternative.

Table 1 Equivalence of HbA1c to blood glucose (most meters measure the plasma glucose)

HbA1c %	Plasma glucose mmol/L	mg/dL	Whole blood glucose mmol/L	mg/dL
5	5.6	103	5.1	92
6	7.6	138	6.9	124
7	9.6	173	8.6	156
8	11.5	208	10.4	188
9	13.5	243	12.2	219
10	15.5	278	13.9	251
11	17.5	314	15.7	283
12	19.5	349	17.4	314

The outcome for control of diabetes needs to be measured in terms of not just biochemical parameters but also the impact on the quality of life of the individual. If a patient is placed on a regimen that they do not like or understand, the outcome is invariably poor glycaemic control. The clinician therefore needs to understand the needs of the patient, for instance a patient with needle phobia may want fewer injections or an insulin pump, whereas a teenage girl may hate the thought of wearing

ADMINISTRATION OF INSULIN

an insulin pump. However, the landmark DCCT study clearly demonstrated that tighter control reduces long-term morbidity from diabetes.

To assess the impact on quality of life one should assess the occurrence of diabetic ketoacidosis and hypoglycaemia (awareness of it and the severity at each clinic visit). Hypoglycaemia in particular impacts on the individual. Fear of undetected nocturnal hypoglycaemia is often the most feared complication for patients and their families. One should also bear in mind the distress that a child/adolescent feels when they have an hypoglycaemic episode in front of their friends and peers. If one suspects non-compliance of insulin, one needs to look beyond medical causes and ask about the psychological impact on the whole family. One should always be aware that the patient may be struggling with other issues outside their diabetes and until such time as one addresses these, the diabetes is often impossible to control.

In the longer term, the aim is to screen for emergence of comorbidities. Controversy still exists with defining the points at which interventions should be introduced in a paediatric age group. Broadly, if there is persistence of any parameter of comorbidity screened such as a raised blood pressure then intervention is recommended. Screening for dyslipidaemia is not yet recommended in the paediatric age group, unlike guidelines for adults, and is a reflection of the lack of evidence in this area.

▷ Further reading

The DCCT Research Group. Adverse events and their association with treatment regimes in the diabetes control and complications trial. *Diabetes Care* 1995;**18**:1415–27.

The DCCT Research Group. Effect of intensive diabetes treatment on the development and progression of long-term complications in adolescents with insulin-dependent diabetes mellitus: Diabetes Control and Complications Trial. *Pediatrics* 1994;**125**:177–88.

Hanas R. *Type 1 Diabetes in Children, Adolescents and Young Adults*, 3rd edn. London: Class Publishing, 2006.

Clinical Practice Consensus Guidelines 2006–2007 of ISPAD. Published in the December 2006 to June 2007 issues of *Pediatric Diabetes*.

▶ Background

Many haematological and non-haematological disorders can affect the bone marrow. In such situations, bone marrow biopsy – aspirate and trephine – will allow quantitative and qualitative assessment. Bone marrow aspirate (collection of a sample of liquid bone marrow) enables morphological assessment of the cellular components while additional samples can be sent for other tests. Bone marrow trephine biopsy (sampling of a small core of bone containing bone marrow) provides a more accurate picture of quantitative changes, bone marrow architecture and bone and stroma abnormalities. On many occasions, bone marrow aspirates and trephine biopsies complement each other necessitating the performance of both procedures. This chapter will only describe bone marrow aspiration.

▷ Indications

A full review and assessment of history, clinical examination and results of relevant investigations should be done to ensure that appropriate indications exist and that adequate and appropriate samples (unilateral/bilateral bone marrow aspirate and/or bone marrow trephine biopsy) have been obtained. The request for a bone marrow aspirate therefore, should be seen as a consultation for full assessment and not a request to carry out a technical procedure.

The material obtained from the bone marrow aspiration biopsy is primarily used to prepare slides for the morphological evaluation of the cellular components. Table 1 lists other tests that can be performed on bone marrow samples and how the information they provide contributes to the diagnosis and management.

Table 1 Tests required on a bone marrow sample and how their interpretation guides diagnosis and management

Tests applied routinely	Haematologist's interpretation: to identify
Morphology on a Romanowsky stained film	Quantitative and morphological abnormalities, revealing leukaemia/lymphoma, solid tumour infiltration, or dysplastic features
Perls' stain for haemosiderin	Abnormal iron inclusions or absent iron stores
Tests applied selectively	
Other cytochemical staining	Nature of infiltrating cells, where the aberrant expression of cell markers is not diagnostic
Immunophenotyping	The subtype of leukaemias, lymphomas and immunodeficiencies
Cytogenetic analysis	The subtype and the prognostic group of leukaemias, lymphomas, solid tumours and myelodysplastic syndromes
Molecular genetic analysis	Cryptic genetic abnormalities, to further identify prognostic groups of leukaemias, lymphomas and myelodysplastic syndromes
Microarrays/gene profiling	A more accurate risk-adapted treatment for leukaemias and lymphomas
Tests for mycobacteria, Leishmania, Histoplasma, or other microorganisms	Causes of pyrexia of unknown origin (PUO)
Culture of colony-forming units	Suspected myeloproliferative disorders
Electron microscopy	Suspected congenital dyserythropoietic anaemia

The commonest indications to perform a bone marrow aspiration are the diagnosis and evaluation of suspected haematological malignancies – leukaemias and lymphomas. A less common indication is the staging evaluation of certain solid tumours in childhood like primitive neuroectodermal tumour (PNET), neuroblastoma, soft tissue sarcomas and Ewing's sarcoma. Rare indications are acquired and congenital bone marrow failure syndromes, myelodysplastic syndrome, suspected histiocytic disorders, immunological disorders, storage disorders and osteopetrosis. Bone marrow aspiration may also be helpful in the investigation of pyrexia of unknown origin (PUO).

Patients with typical features of immune thrombocytopenic purpura, who need no treatment, a bone marrow examination is not required. Consider the procedure if malignancy is suspected or steroid treatment is planned. Bone marrow aspirate is of value in assessing response to treatment after chemotherapy and haemopoietic stem cell transplant.

▷ Contraindications – safety

In experienced hands, bone marrow aspiration is a safe procedure. There are very few contraindications to the procedure. Significant acquired or congenital coagulopathy should be corrected to prevent haemorrhage. In thrombocytopenic patients prolonged local pressure at the puncture site after the procedure is usually sufficient to prevent haemorrhage. It is advisable that the platelet count should be above 20×10^9/L. Sites with overlying skin/soft tissue infection can potentially lead to osteomyelitis by introducing infection into the bone.

▷ Age-related considerations

The posterior ileum is the preferred site for obtaining bone marrow aspirates and biopsies in children of all ages. The anterior ileum is a suitable alternative in older children if it is technically difficult to access the posterior ileum (e.g. severe obesity).

Bone consistency differs in different age groups. Bone consistency during infancy is soft and can be indistinguishable from cartilaginous tissue. Hard bone in an infant with pancytopenia can be associated with osteopetrosis. In contrast the bone of adolescent boys is normally very hard.

Bone marrow aspirate is generally performed under general anaesthesia (GA) or sedation. Local anaesthesia is still used at patient's request or in cases where GA is contraindicated (e.g. large mediastinal mass).

The nature of the procedure needs to be explained to the child and their parents. Appropriate written informed consent is then obtained. Ideally the patient and their parents should also be given appropriate written information.

Pitfalls

- The commonest problem encountered is the failure to obtain bone marrow, the so-called 'dry tap'. This is common in cases of heavy infiltration, aplastic anaemia, previous pelvic irradiation, and rare cases of myelofibrosis. In these cases trephine biopsy for touch preparation and histological staining is indicated. Touch preparations are slides prepared by gently rolling the core bone on to the slide.
- Haemodiluted samples may result from taking large volumes of bone marrow from the same puncture. Haemodilution leads to inadequate material for assessment.
- It is essential that the laboratories that will process the samples be informed of the timing of the procedure. Ensure that the appropriate slides and containers (EDTA/heparin etc.) are available to hand depending on the investigations required. If the patient is enrolled in a

clinical trial, review the protocol to determine the nature of any required bone marrow samples. A number of different types and sizes of bone marrow aspirate needles are commercially available. It is important to be familiar with the type of needle that is available in your institution.

▷ Results and their interpretation

The evaluation of children's bone marrow samples requires a detailed knowledge of the age-specific features of the normal paediatric bone marrow as well as the characteristics of childhood haematological and non-haematological diseases that affect the marrow.

A blood film should be examined as part of the assessment of the bone marrow aspirate.

The report on the bone marrow films should differentiate factual statements from opinion. The factual statement should include the salient clinical and laboratory features. The report should then include the site of aspiration, whether aspiration was easy or difficult, and whether or not bone texture was normal. The body of the report should include an assessment of cellularity and a systematic description of each lineage. The report should include a list of other investigations that have been performed, so that clinical staff are aware of any investigations that are still pending. Finally, the report should have a conclusion in which it is appropriate to express an opinion.

▷ Further reading

Bain BJ. Bone marrow aspiration. *J Clin Pathol* 2001;**54**:657–63.

▶ Subcutaneous injection

Background

Subcutaneous injection is used in circumstances that require slow absorption of medication over several hours. The reason for this is that there is minimal blood flow to fatty tissue, therefore the drug is absorbed into the system at a slower rate. The subcutaneous route may also be used for palliative care pain relief by using a small butterfly needle and syringe driver.

How and where?

Subcutaneous injection is given into the fatty layer underneath the skin. Usually, an extremely fine needle is used so that minimal discomfort is caused and the quantity of medicine administered is also small in volume, usually less that 0.5 mL.

There are several sites that are preferred for subcutaneous injection, including the upper arm, abdomen, upper thigh and lower back. For babies the preferred site is the upper thigh.

Method

- Clean the injection site with an alcohol swab and let the area dry.
- Be careful not to contaminate the needle by touching it with your hands or other surfaces.
- Hold the syringe in one hand like a pencil or a dart in your dominant hand.
- Grasp a skinfold between the thumb and index finger with your free hand.
- Quickly thrust the needle all the way into the skin using a gentle stabbing motion. Insert the needle at a 90 degree angle (Figure 1). However, for small children, and those with little subcutaneous fat on thin skin, you may use a 45 degree angle.
- Release the skin that you are grasping.
- With your free hand, grasp the syringe near its base to stabilise it.

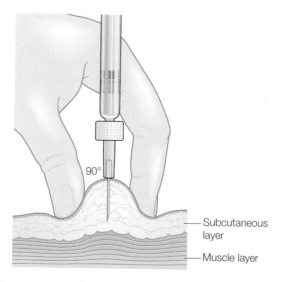

90°

—Subcutaneous layer

—Muscle layer

Figure 1 A subcutaneous injection into the fatty layer of tissue under the skin.

- Gently pull back on the plunger and check for the appearance of blood in the syringe. If blood appears, remove the needle and discard it and start the whole process again. Blood in the syringe means that you may be in a blood vessel, so discard the syringe with medication. Do not inject medication into a blood vessel – the medication is absorbed too rapidly if it is injected there.
- If no blood appears, inject the medication at a slow, steady rate. As the needle is pulled out of the skin, gently press gauze onto the needle insertion site. Pressure over the site while removing the needle prevents skin from pulling back, which may be uncomfortable. A little blood at the site after the needle is removed is of no consequence.

Helpful hints

- It is extremely important to rotate subcutaneous injection sites to maintain the integrity of the skin. Repeated injections in the same spot can cause scarring and hardening of fatty tissue that will interfere with absorption of medication.
- Avoid giving injections in areas that are burned, reddened, inflamed or swollen.

▶ Intramuscular injection

Background

Intramuscular (IM) injection is a method of administering medication deep into muscle tissue. This gives a quicker uptake and absorption of the medication into the patient's system, due to the better blood supply to this tissue mass compared with subcutaneous injection.

Due to the relatively small number of sensory nerves in muscle tissue, IM injection provides a less painful route for administration of irritating drugs.

Needles used for IM injection are longer than those for subcutaneous injection as they must reach deep into the muscle. The gauge of the needle must be appropriate to accommodate viscous solutions and suspensions. The needle length used depends on injection site. Common sites used are the upper arm, outer upper quadrant of the buttocks and the upper thigh. Intramuscular injections should not be administered to areas that are inflamed, oedematous, scarred, have moles or birth marks or any other lesions. They are contraindicated in individuals with coagulopathies or impaired peripheral vascular circulation.

Method

- Clean the injection site with an alcohol swab and let the area dry.
- Be careful not to contaminate the needle by touching it with your hands or other surfaces.
- Hold the syringe in one hand like a pencil or a dart in your dominant hand.
- With your free hand place your index finger on the skin and pull the skin and subcutaneous layer out of alignment with the underlying muscle tissue (Figure 2b).
- Quickly thrust the needle all the way into the skin using a gentle stabbing motion. Insert the needle at a 90 degree angle (Figure 2c). Gently pull back on the plunger and check for the appearance of blood in the syringe. If blood appears, remove the needle, discard it, and start the whole process again. Blood in the syringe means that you may be in a blood vessel, so discard the syringe with medication. Do not inject medication into a blood vessel: the medication is absorbed too rapidly if it is injected there.
- Gently inject the medication and withdraw the needle at a 90 degree angle.
- Remove your finger and let the skin return to the normal position (Figure 2d).

ADMINISTERING MEDICATION

By blocking the needle pathway after an injection, the Z-track technique allows I.M. injection while minimizing the risk of subcutaneous irritation and staining from such drugs as iron dextran. The illustrations below show how to perform a Z-track injection.

Before the procedure begins, the skin, subcutaneous fat, and muscle lie in their normal positions.

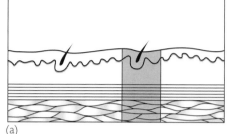

(a)

To begin, place your finger on the skin surface, and pull the skin and subcutaneous layers out of alignment with the underlying muscle. You should move the skin about ½" (1 cm).

(b)

Insert the needle at a 90-degree angle at the site where you initially placed your finger. Inject the drug and withdraw the needle.

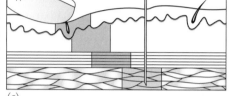

(c)

Finally, remove your finger from the skin surface, allowing the layers to return to their normal positions. The needle track (shown by the dotted line) is now broken at the junction of each tissue layer, trapping the drug in the muscle.

(d)

Figure 2 (a) Normal positions of the skin, subcutaneous tissues and muscle. (b) Place a finger on the skin and pull the skin and subcutaneous tissues by about 1 cm so that they are out of alignment with the muscular layer. (c) Insert needle and inject drug (see text for details). (d) After the finger is removed the tissue layers return to their normal position so that the needle track is interrupted between the layers and the drug is trapped inside the muscle. Redrawn from *Nursing Procedures*, 3rd edn. Lippincott Williams & Wilkins, 2000.

▶ Intravenous injection

The intravenous route is by far the easiest route for administration of medication into the systemic circulation but is associated with the most problems. However, due to the medication being administered directly into the circulation the uptake and absorption of the medicine is immediate. Common drugs administered by this route include antibiotics, antiepileptics and sedatives. This form of administration can also be used for continuous infusion, replacement fluid regimens, transfusion, etc.

The patient will have had a cannula inserted into one of the many veins that are palpable under the subcutaneous tissue layer. Common sites are the back of the hand, lateral wrist, brachial area, saphenous vein and on the top of the foot. Other sites especially in the newborn and infant include veins in the scalp. The medicine to be injected must be prepared aseptically to reduce the risk of contamination. A Luer-lock syringe must be used. Observation of the suspension should demonstrate clarity of substance with no precipitate or foreign bodies. Preparation using a filter needle reduces this risk and is essential in the case of lipid and opaque suspensions, e.g. amphotericin (Abelcet), propofol and prostacycline.

Care of the cannula site is paramount to the safe administration of intravenous medication. The site must be clean and dry, the cannula must be secured well to the skin, and a clear, occlusive dressing applied. The site must be observed while administering medication to check for extravasations, local reaction and leakage from the site.

For administration of more irritant and caustic medicine, central venous access must be gained. This will involve insertion of long lines, triple lumen lines and possibly a Vas Cath. This must be performed by expert practitioners.

▷ Further reading

Elkin MK, Perry AG, Potter PA. *Nursing Interventions and Clinical Skills*. St Louis: Mosby-Year Book Inc, 1996.
Kozier B, Erb G, Blais K, *et al. Techniques in Clinical Nursing*. Canada: Addison-Wesley Nursing, 1993.

▶ Background

The slit lamp provides illumination and high magnification to allow visualisation of the smallest details of the cornea, the anterior chamber, the iris, the lens and the anterior vitreous.

▷ Indications

- To assess symptoms suggestive of disease of the anterior segment of the eye such as irritable red eye, photophobia, eye pain, white pupil or reduced vision. See Table 1 for examples.

Table 1 Symptoms suggestive of anterior eye disease

Symptom	Possible findings	Diagnosis
Persistent irritable eye following minor trauma	Area of cornea fluorescing green with a blue light after instillation of fluorescein eye drops	Corneal abrasion
Redness of the eye in the context of corneal anaesthesia	Staining of the inferior cornea with fluorescein	Exposure keratitis
Severe photophobia in atopic disease	Corneal ulcer usually in superior third of cornea associated with superior peripheral corneal opacities (Trantas dots)	Atopic vernal corneal ulcer
Photophobia, watery discharge, hazy cornea and red eye in irritable infant	Corneal oedema, increased corneal diameter, splits in endothelium of inner surface of cornea	Congenital glaucoma
White pupil	Opacity at level of lens	Cataract
White pupil, premature baby now aged 6 months	Vascularised opacity lying immediately behind the pupil	Total retinal detachment caused by retinopathy of prematurity

- To identify asymptomatic sight-threatening complications of systemic disease, especially juvenile chronic arthritis (JCA). JCA-related uveitis is usually asymptomatic until late in the disease, when irreversible damage with significant risk of blindness may have occurred. The prognosis for vision is closely linked to the severity of clinical signs at the start of treatment. The diagnosis of juvenile chronic arthritis therefore demands prompt slit lamp examination. Before leaving the paediatric clinic, the child's eyes should be examined with a pen torch to look for indications for *urgent* slit lamp examination (Table 2).

Table 2 Indications for urgent slit lamp examination

Findings on examination with a pen torch suspicious of advanced uveitis	Findings on slit lamp examination	Abnormality
Haziness of the cornea	Opacity of the temporal and nasal cornea	Band keratopathy
Irregular small pupil	After mydriatic drops: crenulated pupil margin with pigment deposits on lens and adhesions between iris and lens	Posterior synechiae
Diminished red reflex	Lens opacity	Cataract

- To identify ocular signs that may contribute to the diagnosis of systemic disease. There are numerous systemic conditions in which corneal or other anterior segment signs may contribute to the diagnosis. In some cases completely asymptomatic eye signs may play a key role in reaching an early diagnosis (for examples see Table 3).

Table 3 Asymptomatic eye signs

Suspected condition	Sign on slit lamp examination
Alagille's syndrome	Posterior embryotoxon, i.e. circumferential ridge on the inner surface of the cornea 1–2 mm from the corneoscleral junction
Neurofibromatosis	Lisch nodules, i.e. raised dome-shaped pigmented nodules on the iris
Marfan's syndrome	Wobbling of the iris (iridodonesis) on eye movement
Wilson's disease	Kayser–Fleischer ring, i.e. brownish haze in peripheral cornea
Cystinosis	Fine crystalline deposits throughout the cornea

▷ Equipment and procedure

The standard slit lamp is mounted on a table. The patient rests their chin on a chin rest and brings their forehead forward to a headband. The examiner looks through a binocular microscope focused on structures illuminated by a narrow slit of light. The slit beam provides high contrast illumination. Moreover it provides a cross-sectional view of transparent structures such as the cornea. Sensation of depth in non-transparent structures is enhanced by shadows when the light is shone from one side.

Mechanical linkage between the illuminating arm of the instrument and the microscope keeps the small illuminated area in focus while it is viewed under high magnification. Mechanical linkage between the head rest and the microscope keeps the position of the eye reasonably stable and within range of focus of the microscope. With the portable slit lamp, there is no head rest, so movement between the slit lamp and the child may limit the magnification that can be used.

▷ Different age groups

Slit lamp examination should be possible in children of all ages, although it is often necessary to be persistent, perhaps bringing the child back for a second examination. Small infants may be held on the standard slit lamp in the prone position with the head resting against the forehead band. The vertical height adjustment of most slit lamp tables does not allow preschool children to sit at the slit lamp with their knees under the table. In this situation the child may be able to kneel on the chair to achieve enough height to reach the chin rest, or widely abduct their legs to bring their knees to each side of the slit lamp table rather than under the table. Children with JCA need special consideration because of the extra difficulty children with arthritis may have at positioning themselves at the slit lamp.

Pitfalls

- Failure to position the child's forehead against the headband of the slit lamp is a common cause of being unable to carry out slit lamp examination. The portable slit appears less intimidating but unless the examiner can steady their hand against the child, the magnification that can be used is limited and may not be good enough to detect anterior uveitis.
- Slit lamp examination is not uncomfortable and if the parents understand and explain the procedure to the child and the child has the opportunity to see what is involved, possibly by watching an older sibling or parent being examined, they are usually happy to cooperate. Particularly in JCA, it is unwise to force the child to be examined, since the child's cooperation will be required over years.

▷ Results and their interpretation

- The interpretation of slit lamp examination for symptomatic eye disorders is the province of the ophthalmologist. However, the paediatrician or paediatric specialist nurse should be aware that persistent anterior segment symptoms require further slit lamp examination and a specific diagnosis.

- In **anterior uveitis** cells are seen suspended in the anterior chamber like dust particles illuminated by a sunbeam. The amount of cellular activity is graded from 0 to 4 where +1 or greater is clearly abnormal. The degree of activity is used to gauge the amount of anti-inflammatory treatment required in the short term. Findings such as band keratopathy, posterior synechiae and lens opacity indicate advanced disease. They are key to determining prognosis, long-term management and the role of potentially toxic second line systemic anti-inflammatory agents.

- The interpretation of slit lamp findings that may contribute to the diagnosis of systemic disease depends on knowledge of the prevalence of the findings in healthy and affected children. Posterior embryotoxon is found in some 10 per cent of the normal population, but 80 per cent of patients with Alagille's syndrome. Thus, a finding of posterior embryotoxon contributes to the diagnosis in a child with jaundice of early infancy but by no means guarantees the diagnosis and absence of the sign does not exclude it. Similarly Lisch nodules are found in nearly all adults with neurofibromatosis, but only a third of 2.5-year-olds and only 50 per cent of 5-year-olds. Moreover, they are harder to identify with confidence when they first develop. Thus firm identification of Lisch nodules is more useful than failure to detect them, or uncertain findings in younger children.

▶ Background

Vision is of vital importance to normal infant development. The testing of visual acuity in children is dependent on the child's level of development and assessment of visual acuity always forms part of a comprehensive developmental examination of any child. It is essential to detect and treat ocular abnormalities early to prevent impaired visual development during the first few months of life. For example, if a dense unilateral congenital cataract is not treated within this time then this may result in failure of normal visual development in the affected eye even if the cataract is corrected at a later date.

▷ Indications

Visual acuity testing of children forms part of the UK's child health surveillance programme. All infants born in the UK will have their eyes examined for congenital cataracts as part of the neonatal examination. As part of the child health surveillance, developmental examinations throughout childhood include examination of visual behaviour. On school entry, all children will be offered a visual acuity examination. Apart from the screening tests visual acuity testing should be carried out for the following reasons:

- Parental concerns regarding vision
- Abnormal ocular movements
- Squint
- Systemic disease with a high risk of eye disease, e.g. diabetes
- Prematurity

▷ Affect of age

The methods used to test visual acuity are obviously dependent on the child's developmental age. Once a child is confidently verbal then visual acuity examination becomes easier and more objective. There are many different methods for examining visual acuity in pre-verbal children.

▷ Results and interpretation

- **Red reflex**: It is important to establish, prior to starting any visual acuity tests that both red reflexes are present and there is no evidence of cataract.
- **Fixing and following**: From birth onwards infants preferentially look at faces. By 2–3 weeks a baby should be able to fix on a face and by 6 weeks a baby should consistently be able to fix and follow a face. The baby should be held at arms length away from the tester while moving their face slowly.
- **The spinning test**: When fixing and following can not be demonstrated then this test is used to differentiate between low level vision and blindness. The spinning test relies on the vestibular-ocular reflex. Whilst rotating the infant, nystagmus will occur towards the direction of the rotation. Once the spinning stops the nystagmus should stop over a short period as the baby fixates on the surrounding area. If the nystagmus persists for a long duration then this is suggestive of poor vision.
- **Forced choice preferential looking**: Babies prefer to look at patterned stimulus rather than plain stimulus. The baby is presented at the same time with two cards, one with a patterned stimulus and the other homogeneous but of similar brightness. The examiner is blinded to the location of the patterned card and chooses the most likely location based on the infant's eye movements. The patterned cards will be

changed with increasing spatial frequency until the eye movements indicate no preference between the cards. At this point the level of the infant's visual acuity can be deciphered.

- **Pattern visual evoked potential**: Electrophysiology is a useful means to test vision in the non-verbal child. The test does not require any eye movement as a response. A chequered board with differing sizes is used as the stimulus to the retina and leads are placed over the occipital scalp area looking for an appropriate response. If the child is visually impaired further electrophysiological tests can be carried out to test the different parts of the visual pathway. The electroretinogram (ERG) provides information as to whether the cones and rods are functioning normally. The visual evoked potential can be used to assess the visual pathway in infants and does not require the child to be able to fixate.

- **Cards/charts:** A child's near and distance vision can be accurately tested using different cards/charts. For preschool children the cards used for testing are the Sheridan Gardiner test and Kay cards. There are tests cards for both near and distance vision. The child has to be cognitively able to select matching shapes/letters or pictures. Once a child is able to read, a Snellen chart can be used to test distance vision and the Moorfields reading test or bar-reading test can be used to test near vision.

- **Colour vision**: There are different tools that can be used to test colour vision: Ishihara pseudoisochromatic plates are used to detect red-green colour problems; and Handy–Rand–Rittler plates and Mollon–Reffin test can be used to detect red-green and blue-yellow colour problems.

▷ **Further reading**

Moore A (ed.) *Paediatric Ophthalmology*. London: BMJ Books, 2000.

► Background

The assessment of hearing at an early stage is particularly important as once hearing loss is recognised there may be interventions to improve or even correct it. The impact of poor hearing on development, in particular speech and language acquisition, can be huge, especially in the first few months of life. Language problems can lead to educational difficulties, social and psychological problems.

Assessment of hearing in children is the responsibility of many health professionals including hearing screeners, audiologists, health visitors, school nurses, teachers, general practitioners, paediatricians and ear, nose and throat surgeons. We must also remember the role of parents and carers, who are sometimes the first to identify concerns.

Any child found to have hearing difficulties or hearing loss should be managed by a multidisciplinary team, whose focus is on the medical, educational, developmental, social and psychological needs of the child and their family.

▷ Indications

The indications for hearing testing can be divided into three categories:

- routine hearing screening
- targeted screening
- symptoms attributable to hearing loss

▷ Routine hearing screening tests

- With the introduction of the newborn hearing screening programme every baby should undergo a hearing check within the first few weeks of life. This is an otoacoustic emissions test. If the baby does not pass this test a second screening test, an auditory brainstem response, can be performed.
- At approximately 8 months of age a distraction test will be performed by the health visitor.
- Finally, at school entry a modified pure tone audiometry test will be carried out. Most significant hearing difficulties will have been picked up by this time, but mild, unilateral or progressive hearing problems may be identified.

▷ Targeted screening

Targeted screening is instigated where there is a family history of a parent with childhood sensorineural deafness or where specific medical problems are known to increase the risk of hearing loss. There are both congenital and acquired conditions that require monitoring of hearing.

Children born with a congenital infection or conditions that increase the risk of middle ear problems, such as Down's syndrome or craniofacial abnormalities, will be regularly screened and tested for hearing loss. The exact frequency of review will depend on local policies. Acquired problems requiring follow-up hearing tests include the following:

- hyperbilirubinaemia requiring exchange transfusion
- meningitis
- severe head injury
- prolonged intensive care
- birth weight less than 1500 g
- ototoxic drugs where levels have exceeded the normal therapeutic range

▷ Symptomatic concerns

The significance of parental observations cannot be stressed highly enough and parents should be encouraged to observe their child's reaction to sounds and also making noises. As part of the newborn screening programme parents are provided with a checklist for reaction to and making sounds. This provides even the inexperienced parent with information as to what is expected in their child from birth to 36 months of age. If parents feel that their child is not meeting these targets they can seek advice from their health visitor or general practitioner. School teachers, often with their wealth of experience, are also crucial in identifying potential problems and should be listened to. Some of the specific problems that may arise in a child with hearing problems are as follows:

- speech delay
- pronunciation difficulties
- a child that talks loudly or listens to loud volume music/television
- educational difficulties, especially in the context of known glue ear
- behavioural difficulties, including anger, frustration or communication problems
- withdrawal and social isolation

▷ Types of hearing tests

Table 1 summarises the different hearing tests, what they are assessing, the equipment needed and their potential pitfalls. As with all patient-centred tests, failure to instruct the patient correctly or indeed to take into account the need for language interpretation will give unreliable results. Also equipment malfunction or failure to regularly check and maintain instrumentation will give false outcomes.

Age considerations

It is vital to think about both the child's age and developmental status in the context of the choice of hearing testing. Matching the appropriate test to the child will help with their compliance and therefore the diagnostic yield.

Results and interpretation

- **Otoacoustic emissions**: in the healthy cochlea, vibration of the hair cells in response to noise generates acoustic energy, known as otoacoustic emissions. If in response to the noise stimulus a strong response is produced it is normal. If there is no response or a dampened response, further tests are needed to assess inner ear function and the auditory pathway. This would usually be an auditory brainstem response test.
- **Auditory brainstem response**: after the auditory stimuli, normally a series of clicks, is generated, the latencies (in milliseconds) and amplitude (in microvolts) of the waves produced are recorded. Waves I and II are generated from the eighth cranial nerve and III–V from the brainstem and midbrain. This allows identification of the different parts of the auditory pathway involved. Measurements are compared against normal ranges for age and sex. A conductive hearing loss would show prolonged latencies of all waves. A sensorineural hearing loss may show prolonged latencies and reduced amplitude of waves or even an absence of waves.
- **Distraction testing**: this screening test is used to assess the child's response to high and low frequency sound. A positive response and pass is indicated by a clear turn of the head to the sound at a 30 decibel (dB) level. This would imply the absence of significant hearing loss. Failure to satisfy these criteria includes failure to turn the head, poor localisation of the sound or incorrect localisation of the sound. In this situation referral for formal audiological assessment is required.

Table I Overview of hearing tests

Test/purpose	Equipment	False positives	False negatives
Otoacoustic emissions Assesses inner ear cochlear (specifically hair cells)	• Soft tipped earpiece probe compromising sound emitter and microphone • Computer with software	• Fluid or debris in ear canal • Middle ear pathology • Restless baby • Noisy environment	• Computer failure • Test does not evaluate or exclude auditory neuropathy
Auditory brainstem response Assesses inner ear, auditory nerve pathway and brainstem	• Ear probe or headphones with sound emitter • Scalp electrodes • Computer with software	• Outer ear obstruction or middle ear pathology • Restless baby/uncooperative child • Noisy environment or electrical interference	• Computer failure
Distraction testing Assesses low and high frequency hearing	• Voice, rattles and warblers • Sound protected room	• Physically unable to sit, balance or turn to noise • Uncooperative or bored child • Noisy environment	• Person with child reacts to distractions • No pauses or variation in timing of noises • Assessor in child's field of vision • No pauses or variation in timing of
Pure tone audiometry Assesses both conductive and sensorineural hearing	• Headphones and bone vibrator • Computer producing pure tones 125–8000 Hz • Trained operator using bracketing technique • Sound protected room	• Poorly placed headphone • Noisy environment • Operator failure	• Operator failure stimulus delivered
Impedance testing (tympanometry) Measures compliance of the tympanic membrane	• Probe comprising three channels for sound delivery, pressure delivery and microphone • Computer with software	• Inadequate seal around probe • Perforated ear drum	• Computer failure
Electrocochleography Assesses cochlear and VIIIth cranial nerve	• Ear probe or needle probe through tympanic membrane • Reference surface electrodes • Computer software	• Problems with equipment and computer software • Lack of reliable normal results	• Problems with equipment and computer software • Lack of reliable normal results

HEARING TESTING

- **Pure tone audiometry**: this measures the threshold level of hearing that is heard at different frequencies for both air and bone conduction. This is recorded as the decibel hearing level for that frequency. Symbols are used to represent the different thresholds tested. An **O** represents the right air conduction threshold, **X** the left air conduction threshold, [the right bone conduction threshold and] the left bone conduction threshold. A normal audiogram will usually show a hearing threshold of 0–20 dB at frequencies of 125–8000 Hertz. A conductive hearing loss, such as glue ear, will show an increase in the hearing threshold across all frequencies for air conduction alone. Bone conduction remains normal. A sensorineural loss will show an increase in the hearing threshold for both air and bone conduction. Thresholds in hearing loss can be considered as mild (20–40 dB), moderate (40–60 dB), severe (60–80 dB) and profound (greater than 80 dB).
- **Impedance testing**: results are expressed as compliance plotted against pressure. A normal trace will show a tympanometric peak, representing maximum flow of acoustic energy, at a zero pressure, i.e. when the pressure in the external ear canal is the same as the middle ear pressure. A flattened trace with a normal canal volume usually signifies the presence of fluid behind the tympanic membrane. With eustachian tube dysfunction the peak wave form is at a negative pressure rather than at zero.
- **Electrocochleography**: this is a variant of the auditory brainstem response where the recording electrode is placed as close as practically possible to the cochlea. It is a method for recording the electrical potentials of the cochlea. This involves measurement of the summating potential, reflecting hair cell activity, and the compound action potential of the auditory nerve. Interpretation is specialised and beyond the realms of this text but it is used to diagnose Ménière's disease and swelling of the inner ear and can also be used for intraoperative monitoring.

▷ Further reading

Roland NJ, McRae RDR, McCombe AW. *Key Topics in Otolaryngology*, 2nd edn. London: Taylor & Francis, 2001.